BEYOND YIN AND YANG
HOW ACUPUNCTURE REALLY WORKS

BEYOND YIN AND YANG
HOW ACUPUNCTURE REALLY WORKS

By

GEORGE A. ULETT, M.D., Ph.D.
Clinical Professor of Psychiatry
University of Missouri School of Medicine

Associate Director for Policy
Missouri Institute of Mental Health
and
Director of Department of Psychiatry
Deaconess Hospital
St. Louis, MO

WARREN H. GREEN, INC.
St. Louis, Missouri, U.S.A.

Published by

WARREN H. GREEN, INC.
8356 Olive Boulevard
Saint Louis, Missouri, 63132 U.S.A.

© 1992 by WARREN H. GREEN, INC.

ISBN No. 0-87527-490-0

2nd Printing 1998

Printed in the United States of America

INTRODUCTION

There is an old Chinese proverb which states, "one generation opens the road upon which another generation travels". It is a tribute to those ancient Chinese physicians that some of the acupuncture points they selected, by trial and error, coincide with now recognized anatomical structures. Many of their clinical observations have direct pertinence to current medical concepts. Due, however, to the almost non-existent scientific knowledge of that time, explanations were couched in fanciful metaphysical and numerological terms. Since then, with the passing of 3000 years, medical science has made great strides. Building upon these early empirical observations, neuroscientists have, in this decade of the brain, opened new vistas in our understanding of central nervous system mechanisms.

Acupuncture, viewed in historical perspective, is an important stone in the structure of the medical specialty of Algology, for acupuncture's principal use is in the treatment of pain. The World Health Organization has stated that it is used by well over one third of the world's population.

Acupuncture is essentially a treatment based upon actions of the nervous system. One could say that although nervous structures were unknown to them, the early Chinese physicians were the first to describe the action of the Central Nervous system. Chhi is, in reality, the energy of the nervous impulse. Useful acupuncture points are areas that are heavily innervated by motor and sensory nerve terminals or points adjacent to major nerve tracts. The meridians are actually a primitive analogy of nerve pathways.

It is enigmatic that today thousands of acupuncturists, including physicians who should know better, are, through reasons of custom, ignorance or design, practicing the kind of acupuncture that is based upon centuries old, metaphysical theories. Such acupuncturists select their points for stimulation by means of pulse diagnosis, outmoded theories of disease causation, or cabalistic formulae. Persons using such techniques of acupuncture are carrying on their treatments apparently oblivious to the fact that the meridian theory is a myth and that modern acupuncture, as practiced by scientifically trained physicians today in China and elsewhere, can now be a treatment based on factual rather than fanciful ideas.

Ten years have passed since I wrote *Principles and Practice of Physiologic Acupuncture*. It is time to revise that book and mention some of the new discoveries that have produced evidence to strengthen ideas earlier presented. As the term "Physiologic acupuncture," appeared simply to add another type of treatment to the over 125 varieties of acupuncture that now exist, it was decided to select a new title. The title, *Beyond Yin and Yang*, was chosen to challenge and present an alternative to persons who are now practicing a type of acupuncture based upon mystical concepts.

No disparagement is intended to those intuitive, ancient physicians who created the original methods of traditional acupuncture, nor to all those around the world who have, in spite of criticism from the medical establishment, steadfastly extolled the value of acupuncture as a useful form of treatment. The purpose of this book is rather to present current scientific evidence indicating the common physiological basis that underlies all of these forms of acupuncture treatments. This book will present a means to amplify the opportunity for successful treatment by using those principles from neurophysiology that, when properly applied, can serve to strengthen the acupuncture response. What is presented is therefore not a new or another form of acupuncture. It is rather an exposition of today's knowledge. Hopefully, it will serve to render acupuncture palatable to scientific allopathic medicine and to present the factual basis for an approval of this physiologically based method of treatment. Such an understanding is now needed by third party payers and by state licensing bodies. It is hoped that this book will find its way to the shelves of medical school libraries where the next generation of physicians can learn a simple useful method of patient treatment and become interested in seeking answers to the many questions about acupuncture that still remain.

The ideas in this book have come from many sources. They have been gathered from several trips to China, Japan, Hong Kong, Scandinavia and elsewhere. The list of references reveals many of these names but I would be remiss if I did not mention some personal contacts with leaders in the field whose ideas have been important in preparing this manuscript. My love of magic has taught me that all seeming miracles have ordinary explanations. The directions taken by my interest in acupuncture and chronic pain can be traced to certain prominent mentors who were important influences in my professional training. To them I owe a tremendous debt for imbuing in me an eclecticism that has led me on a continual search for the physiological basis of behavioral events. Some of these important persons are: Calvin Stone, Stanford University Dept. of Psychology, who strongly urged me to combine physiology with my interest in psychology; Robert Dow, my respected professor of neuro-anatomy and neuro-physiology; Raymond Adams who coached me in obtaining neurological knowledge that has been necessary for understanding clinical manifestations of pain; Edwin Gildea who fostered an eclectic approach to psychiatry; Kodo Senshu of Tokyo who first convinced me that acupuncture really works and Ji-

Sheng Han, Beijing, upon whose scientific investigations I have leaned heavily for much of this book. My deep appreciation goes to many others including, Felix Mann, London, England; H.C. Wen, Hong Kong; Pierre Nogier, Lyon, France; C.C. Chung, Taiwan; Song Ping Han, St. Louis; Pacita Dee, whose father brought acupuncture to Manila and who developed drawings for the first edition of this book, Sam Parwatikar, John Stern, Marge Brown, Bernd and Monica Saletu, and Ivan Sletten who participated with me in our first research efforts on acupuncture, Esther Schulz who typed and edited many pages of manuscript, Warren Green, a great editor, Jude McKay responsible for cover designs and above all, Pearl C. Ulett, M.D., my faithful wife, born in Suining, Szechuan Province China who was responsible for my interest and love of all things Chinese.

TABLE OF CONTENTS

BEYOND YIN AND YANG
HOW ACUPUNCTURE REALLY WORKS

Chapter I

THE BEGINNINGS: METAPHYSICAL EXPLANATIONS OF ANCIENT CHINESE ACUPUNCTURE

In order to understand the origins of modern scientific acupuncture and to comprehend the writings of the great majority of acupuncturists who still practice according to the outmoded, pre-scientific concepts of "meridian theory," it is well at this point to take an historical look at acupuncture origins. For, as Chairman Mao proclaimed, "ancient Chinese medicine is truly a veritable storehouse" from which has developed much that is useful to modern medicine.

The theories and terminology of Chinese medicine derive from the *Nei Ching* (1) a centuries old medical manuscript. Traditional acupuncture is based upon concepts of "energetic medicine" (2) a belief that there is a continuous generation and flow of energy (chhi, life force) throughout the body. This force is believed to have two polarities, Yin and Yang. When the flow of these energies is felt to be in balance, a state of health exists. Illness occurs when they are out of balance. These energies travel through the body over 12 major channels (meridians), each linked to a particular organ or body function. On each meridian there exist numerous acupuncture points at each of which it is taught that the flow of energy is close to the surface and can be influenced by the insertions and manipulation of needles. Such needling (pique) can either strengthen (tonify) deficient energy in a given organ/system or weaken (disperse) excess energy.

A traditional acupuncturist must determine through a palpation of the 12 radial pulses which meridian is deficient in energy. Such pulse diagnosis is felt to be the means for detecting illness before actual symptoms of disease occur (3). Thus acupuncture is used to correct Yin/Yang balance and prevent illness. When symptoms of disease are already present, it is thought that the existing pain and symptoms cause such a disturbance of body equilibrium that pulse diagnosis is of little use and the treatment is then placed on an inferior basis requiring only the placement of needles according to a "set formula" of points. Each of these formulae is specific for a particular illness. Once the illness has been corrected a master of acupuncture can then discern from the pulse which meridian imbalance has caused the illness and in this manner determine the proper placement of the needles to prevent further malfunction.

3

The theoretical basis for treatment by acupunture was developed from a consideration of the interrelationship of five elements or essential forces, each of which was related to a pair of organs. One set of organs was "hollow" (fu: small intestine, gall bladder, stomach, colon and urinary bladder). The other set was "solid" (tsang: heart, liver, spleen, lungs and kidney), later, "triple heater" and "pericardium" concepts were added respectively to the two groups, thus raising the number of organs to 12 in order to match the 12 meridians.

An elaborate set of rules governed the selection of treatment points utilizing not only a formula relating these elements (meridians/organs) in terms of dominance and submission, but as well the relationship of the elements to other cosmic forces e.g., nature, color, sounds etc. Lists of acupuncture points to be used were formulated in terms of their relationship to various cosmic forces and the waxing and waning of Yin and Yang strength at different times of the day.

The complexity of the metaphysical theory is such that it is said a lifetime is required to master the total system held as a closely guarded secret by masters of acupuncture or passed on within families from father to son. Inherent in the whole complex approach lies the concept of "balancing energies"," or bringing forces into harmony. Hence, the same point is felt to be of use to either increase or decrease a given function, depending upon the state of energy balance in the body at the time and the manner of stimulation used.

Acupuncture is but one part of traditional Chinese medicine The use of herbs and other types of physical manipulation such as diet are equally important. The theoretical basis of Chinese medicine was built around attempts to explain health, illness and man's relationship to the universe at a time prior to recorded history. There was then but the barest knowledge of anatomy , practically no idea of physiology and in China, as elsewhere in the world, concepts of life, health and illness were based upon philosophic ideas, superstition and religion. Thus acupuncture theory is but a reflection of the primitive beliefs of that period.

In keeping with Taoistic philosophy, man was thought to be a micro-cosmic reflection of the cosmos. The central, single world force, perfect whole or Tao was the Yin/Yang consisting of two elements Yin and Yang. These two opposing complimentary forces each stood for one of paired elements. All manner of opposites could be classified as being either Yang or Yin in nature (e.g., male/female, heaven/earth, powerful/weak, fire/water, well/sick, etc.).

Yin/Yang is traditionally diagrammed as a circle containing its two components. Starting at either pole and following the center "S" curve as one force increases the other complimentary force wanes. Throughout Chinese medical literature there is often described a tripartition of Yin and Yang. Thus in Figure 1, from bottom to top (right) Yang can be seen to progress from minor Yang through splendor Yang to major Yang, while from top to bottom (left), Yin progresses from minor Yin, through shrinking Yin, to major Yin. It can also be seen centrally there is some small amount of Yin in Yang and Yang in Yin.

In traditional Chinese medicine whole man is the Yin/Yang. The Yin and Yang are two life forces which must be kept in harmonious balance for perfect health. Illness occurs when this balance is disturbed. There are Yin illnesses and Yang illnesses, Yin foods, and Yang foods, herbal medicines to strengthen Yin and herbal medicines to strengthen Yang. In acupuncture there is, therefore a major concern with needling procedures to balance Yin or Yang should either force be deemed weak or in excess.

Second only in importance to Yin and Yang was an understanding of the five evolutive phases (wu shing), of the translated "five element theory." This concept was formulated by Tsou Yen who lived between 350-270 B.C. Like much of Chinese medical theory, the "wu shing:" fire, earth, metal, wood and water, refers not to static elements, like a primitive periodic table, but rather to energetic qualities that are evolving, expanding and contracting within a time frame.

In our brief attempt here to grasp some fundamentals of a vast and complex metaphysical philosophy, we must conceive of an evolution of forces within the human body that is linked to the changing forces of nature. The optimal times for treating various diseases is based upon the time of day at which energy is thought to peak within various organ systems.

In keeping with the microcosmic nature of man, the doctrines and practice of acupuncture needling must in some ways depend upon not only the hour of the day, but as well, upon the season of the year and the position of the moon. Thus, the importance of numerological and astrological concepts for Chinese medicine. Chinese physicians were concerned with the whole man, long predating Western concepts of psychosomatic medicine. Thus, the five evolutive phases are concerned not only with the condition of the physical disease but also with a description of the patient's emotional state as well.

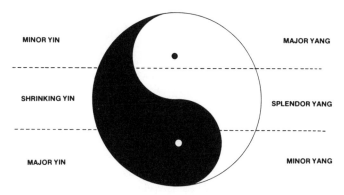

Figure 1. The waxing and waning of Yin and Yang.

In the science of Yin/Yang cycles it was felt that no life, no growth, nor recovery from illness could come without the cooperation of both heavenly and earthly powers. In this system the five elements operated from the heavens, while six "chhi," or life energies derived from earth. There existed the conviction that man was not isolated from nature, thus cyclic astronomical, meteorological, climactic and epidemiological factors were important for physical processes of health and disease.

The five elements became integrated into Yin/Yang theory as wood (Yang minor), fire (Yang major), metal (Yin minor) and water (Yin major). In ancient sections of the *Nei Ching*, the fifth or central evolutive phase, earth, is moved to a position between fire and metal where it has since remained in classical tradition (Fig. 2). The various organs are believed to relate to or function within this traditional framework.

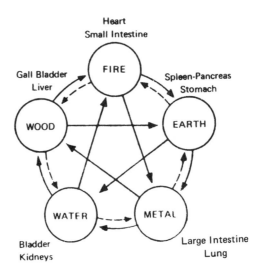

Figure 2. Showing the interaction of the five essences and how they may influence one another. Clockwise rotation is the engendering (strengthening) sheng cycle. Counterclockwise is the overcoming (weakening) ko cycle.

In the therapeutic formulation of Chinese medicine, the influence of one organ system upon other organ systems is determined by the relationship of the five evolutive phases to each other. The "Law of Wu Hing," illustrated in Table I, gives the formulae for treatment through the action of one system on another once it has been determined which of the five elements requires either stimulation or sedation. The so-called "productive sequence," (wu or sheng cycle), conceives of each evolutive phase (element), as the product or "child" (tzo), of each preceding phase (element), which is considered as it's "mother" (mu). In the sheng cycle the element to be treated is determined by selection in clockwise rotation. Similarly, the "checking" or ko sequence, is described in which each evolutive phase (element), is considered as though checking the preceding element. Here, the selection of the element to be treated is viewed as seen in a counter-clockwise rotation. An example of the need for treatment might be as follows: if the energy at a given position has become redundant its qualities are believed to overpower positions that are functionally connected with it. Under these conditions the checking "ko" function becomes a violation of the "wu" sequence, thus producing dysfunction in the corresponding organ or bodily system. Under normal conditions the "productive" and "checking" energetic forces are presumed to act in such fashion as to maintain harmonious balance of function within the organism.

A consideration of the 12 meridians and the requirement of symmetry in pulse diagnosis seemed to dictate the need for six pairs of organs in relation to the five elements Thus we find in the completed diagram (Fig. 3), that fire has been divided into two parts; the heart prince (heart and small intestine) and the heart minister (pericardium and triple warmer). The triple warmer represents three hypothetical spaces in the abdominal cavity concerned with the creation of energy.

For a time we will leave this discussion of the five evolutive phases to return again after a discussion of Chinese pulse diagnosis.

TABLE 1

DOCTRINE OF THE FIVE ELEMENTS. "THE LAW OF WU HING"

Illustrating How These Elements Exercise an
Influence One Upon the Other

THE SHENG CYCLE

FIRE engenders EARTH
EARTH engenders METAL
METAL engenders WATER
WATER engenders WOOD
WOOD engenders FIRE

THE KO CYCLE

FIRE overcomes METAL by melting
METAL overcomes WOOD by cutting
WOOD overcomes EARTH by covering
EARTH overcomes WATER by damming
WATER overcomes FIRE by extinguishing

SPHYGMOLOGY (PULSE DIAGNOSIS) It is of interest that the Chinese conceived the idea of circulation of the blood 200 years B.C., almost two thousand years ago. Blood circulation was formulated in the West by Harvey, 1628 A.D. The early Chinese physicians held that there were two systems of circulation in the body. One was for the blood (mo), concerned with Yin forces. The other was a vaporous life force (chhi). It was a Yang force circulating in the sinarteries (acupuncture meridian tracts). Both mo and chhi had a dual origin partly from nutritional sources and partly inherited from Yin (maternal) and Yang (paternal) influences. According to Chinese medicine, under conditions of normal health all parts of the body are supplied with essential elements to replace metabolic loss and to effect repair by the systems of circulation. Any interference with these resulted in diseases requiring acupuncture, moxibustion or herbs to restore the proper Yin/Yang balance.

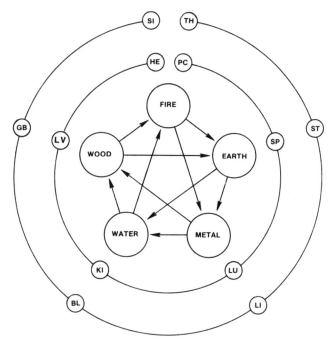

Figure 3. Illustrates the addition of the pericardium (PC) and the triple heaters (TH) to the fire position. This increases the number of organ postions around the five element diagram from 5 to 6 thus permitting concordance with the twelve meridians. Organs shown on the innermost circle are solid (Yin) organs. Those on the outer circle are hollow (Yang) organs.

The *Nei-Ching* dictated that the pulse should be studied during the early morning hours (3 a.m. to 9 a.m.), when the "Yin is immobile and Yang not yet gone from the body." The patient should be fasting with bladder and stomach empty. "At this moment only are blood and energy calm." Such pulse diagnosis was an essential part of Chinese medical practice. It was felt that the radial pulses of the two wrists each provided a reflection of six of the twelve bodily systems indicating the Yin/Yang balance or state of health in each (Fig. 4).

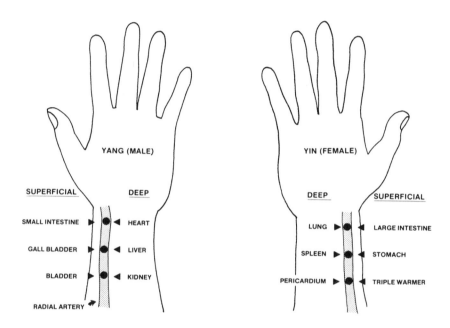

Figure 4. Location of the twelve pulses in relationship to the energy flow to be detected as reflected from the twelve meridians. Interaction between the left and right hand pulses is known as the husband-wife law. Thus the husband may rule the wife but that relationship can be "put in danger" by the wife.

To properly palpate the pulse three fingers (index, middle and ring), are placed upon the radial artery on the radial side of the wrist where the fingers can palpate the artery directly against the radius. The middle finger rests on the bony radial prominence with the index and ring finger palpating the "sun and chhia" sites distally and proximally respectively. There is also a deep and superficial palpation by each of the three fingers. Each pulse is supposed to transmit special information about a specific bodily system. It will be noted that the deep pulses reflect the tsang, (solid) organs, and the superficial pulses, the fu, (hollow) organs. Physicians, well trained in pulse diagnosis, claim to be able to differentiate some 28 qualities of pulse (Fig. 5). Skilled pulse diagnosticians have the reputation for accurate estimation of prognosis in critically ill cases by means of seven "fatal" pulses, e.g., "rolling peas under the finger" (terminal peritonitis), a "feather brushing the cheek" (terminal pulmonary tuberculosis), "movements of a tadpole" (auricular fibrillation), "snapping of a violin's taut string" (hypertensive nephritis), etc. In order to properly assess the pulse the physician must first compose himself in silence, develop his own respiratory rate as normal and count the pulse beats in relation to his own breathing, i.e., four beats of the pulse to each single respiration as a normal baseline.

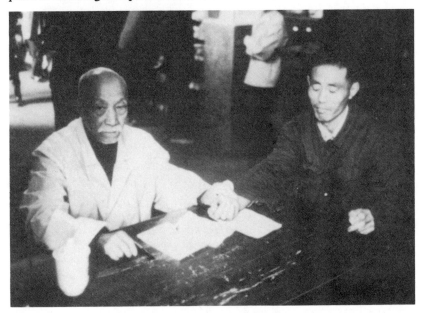

Figure 5. Traditional pulse diagnosis in an herb store in Wuhan, Peoples Republic of China, November, 1980.

The twelve pulses relate to the twelve bodily systems, tsang (Yin) and fu (Yang) organs and as well to the five elements (evolutive phases). This interrelationship determines which organ system needs to be stimulated or calmed in order to restore a harmonic balance to the total system. If, for example, the pulse representing lung (metal-air) was found deficient, one might stimulate spleen (earth) to bring about correction. With the complex interactions described, the same result might be accomplished by acting upon fire (pericardium) or kidney (water). Thus, one can begin to see the multitude of interactions that can be developed with such a complex metaphysical formulation. The rules for determination of the proper point seem almost endless .It is understandable how a vast number of inconsistencies will be found as one reads the voluminous literature that has accumulated on acupuncture through the centuries.

In considering the causation of illness it has been important to recognize the nature and timing of the energy forces circulating within the body. Thus, mo (Yin) and chhi (Yang) were felt to circle endlessly, making 50 revolutions each day and night of twelve double hours. In addition, the ebb and flow of energy in the organ systems followed the clock in such fashion that energy peaked in each system at a given time of the day or night. There thus appeared certain times most effective for the treatment of each afflicted organ/system. To ignore this time-sequenced, hoary cycle was to impair the likelihood of curing the illness.

The theoretical foundations of Chinese medicine thus far summarized form the basis for a therapeutic approach that involves far more than acupuncture. An even larger part of the physician's armamentarium was herbology. A knowledge of the medicinal value of plants was early developed in the Chinese pharmacopia. In the year 1000 there were 1000 herbs classified and available to the treating physician. To each of these herbs was attached, apart from any effect on special organs or systems, the characteristic of Yin or Yang, thus indicating its ability to either stimulate or sedate given meridian functions.

Various colors, sounds, water, music and specific types of food had their representation of equivalence in the five essences, each with specific Yin or Yang effect. From such list, changes in life style or diet would be recommended for their beneficial influence upon the life of the individual. This was, indeed, the epitome of holistic medicine, as the advice given for climate, foods, etc., was designed to prevent as well as to cure. It is said that at one period in Chinese medical history the physician was paid only as long as the patient remained well. With the onset of disease payment ceased, to be resumed only when the physician had accomplished remission from the illness.

Early in the development of Chinese medical history detailed consideration was given to the specific means for conducting energy through the body. The *Huang Ti Nei Ching* (Yellow Emperor's Manual of Corporal Medicine), states that in the section known as the *Su Wen*, blood vessels are to be recognized in the body. In the *Ling Shu* section it was stated that the Yin chhi travels within the blood vassals (mo), while the Yang chhi (wei) travels outside of them. It was with this latter system of conduits that the portion of the *Nei Ching*, known as the *Chen Ching (Manual of the Needles)* was concerned and laid down the first description of points. These points were located on the main channels (acu-tracts or ching). Each has at least one junction (acu-junction or lo) where it connects with one or more neighboring tracts through short branches (lo-mo). This system of ching-lo acupuncture tracts or meridians) is an invisible one but was presumed to run in the subcutaneous tissues of the body. Upon the ching-lo (meridians) are located the acupuncture points (hsueh). The stimulation of these points by needles, pressure, moxibustion or otherwise is felt to influence the flow of chhi through these tracts in such a way as to augment (tonify), or decrease (sedate). and thus reestablish the harmonious Yin/Yang balance.

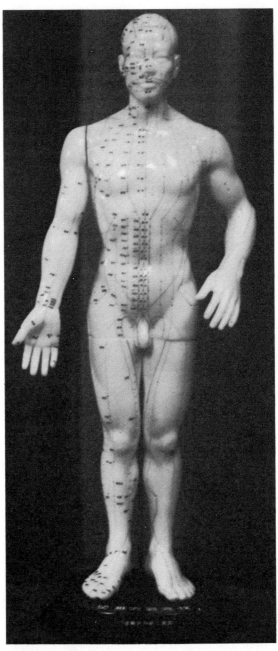

Figure 6. Plastic mannequin used for teaching traditional acupuncture points.

There are described twelve major paired regulatory tracts and eight auxiliary tracts, two of which are unpaired and regulatory, tu mo (governing vessel), and jen mo (conception vessel), and six are connecting. Circulation through the twelve main tracts conforms to the Yin/Yang cycle. The twelve regular paired meridians are universally used by acupuncturists as "road maps" for the location of acupuncture points (Fig. 6). As these acu-tracts have no real anatomical basis, their use to the acupuncturist can be compared to the use of longitude and latitude familiar to the geographer. The eight auxiliary tracts differ in importance and frequency of use by acupuncturists. Tu-mo and jen-mo are the only ones which have acupuncture points of their own and are regularly used along with the twelve paired meridians. The others interact with the twelve regular tracts and their acupuncture points occur at such junctions and are identical with those of the interacting tracts. One of these, known as the great acu-junction of the spleen, is identical with the ta-pao (spleen point 21) and has, because of its importance, been at times designated as a 15th regulatory meridian.

Besides the above, there are twelve ching chin interconnecting neuromuscular tracts. As in ancient Greek anatomy, little distinction was made between tendons, muscles and nerves. The designation of these tracts is similarly unclear. They are thought to pass more superficially than the twelve regular meridians, originating from the tips of the four extremities and passing toward the head, but without any relationship to the viscera. They have no specific points but were commonly treated with heat or with cauterizing needles at the site of any muscular pain.

According to ancient Chinese concepts, the acupuncture points were holes in the body for the passage of energy or at least areas where the energy passed close to the surface and could thus be readily influenced. The Chinese term for acupuncture point, "hsueh," means cave, or hollow and, indeed, many of the points are described as a slight depression that is felt in the subcutaneous tissue. During the course of some illnesses, certain of these points may become tender to palpation, and hence some have been designated, "pressure points." At other times they may be felt as fibrositic nodules beneath the skin, thus coincident with the modern concept of "trigger points." The Chinese called these "Ah Shi" (Oh Yes), points as the patient so replied when asked if the point was tender upon palpation.

The number of recognized acupuncture points has varied over time and with different authors. The named points on the regularly used 14 channels total 361. They are mirror-images, duplicated on both sides of the body except for the 51 points on the midline channels. This brings the total to 671 points (Fig. 7, a,b,c). At this writing, there are some 63 extra meridian points (chhi hsueh), commonly used which are not located on any of the meridians. Another 168 points have been described in the ear called "fan ying tien," and each related to some particular viscera or portion of the body.

While the above are the commonly accepted points, there are, in addition, "private" points discussed and used in their practice by individual acupuncturists. With the growth of acupuncture analgesia for surgery, trial and error experimentation has yielded other points that seem useful for operative procedures and thus today the number of points used in acupuncture may well be over 1000.

Some classes of points are commonly referred to as having specific therapeutic application. These include: points having strong influence over the relationship of meridians to organ functions; tsing points (tips of fingers and toes); yung points (base of fingers and toes); yu points (hands and feet); ching points (wrists and ankles); and wo points (elbows and knees).

Other points with designated therapeutic importance include: points of origin (source or yuan points) for treating dysfunction of that specific organ system; points of anastomosis (lo points), where Yin and Yang meridians meet; points of accumulation (hsi points) useful in treating chronic disease; points of relationship between ventral and dorsal meridians (mo and shu points) thought to have a mutual influence on visceral organs; and points of convergence (wei points), useful in treating illnesses of different types of tissue, viscera and energy. There are, in addition, special points which connect the points of the twelve paired meridians with the eight auxiliary meridians.

Each acupuncture point is carefully described in terms of its surface anatomical location. Their identification is dependent upon local landmarks of the body such as bony tubercles, the nipples, depressions in muscular structure etc. For the location of points away from such landmarks, a system of body measurement was developed. This allows for differences in body size. The unit of self measurement is known as the "cun," "pouce," or "body inch." This is the distance between two folds of the middle phalanx of the middle finger when in the bent position. This body inch is subdivided into 10 lesser units termed "fen." Each point has a designated usefulness for the treatment of some type of illness or symptom. Descriptions of these may be found in the many texts on the subject. While most authors agree quite well on the descriptions for the location of points, there is wide variance as to their therapeutic use.

EAR ACUPUNCTURE (AURICULOTHERAPY). The ear has long been used as an area for treatment in traditional acupuncture. Several chapters of the *Nei Ching* make reference to the six Yang meridians as passing through the ear. Later writings state that all twelve meridians are joined in the ear. The *Nei Ching* also refers to the ear as useful in diagnosing afflictions of the kidney. From the 5th century A.D., acupuncture of the ear was mentioned in the treatment of many diseases. In 1957, the French physician and acupuncturist, Paul Nogier, reported studies relating the ear to other parts of the body. His teachings have served to popularize the subspecialty of auriculotherapy.(4).

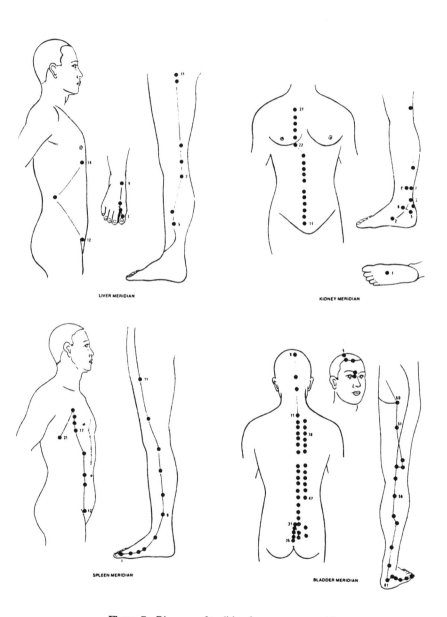

Figure 7a. Diagrams of traditional acupuncture meridians.

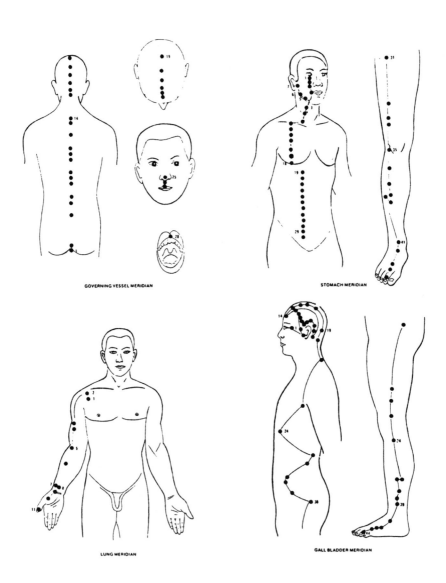

Figure 7b. Diagrams of traditional acupuncture meridians.

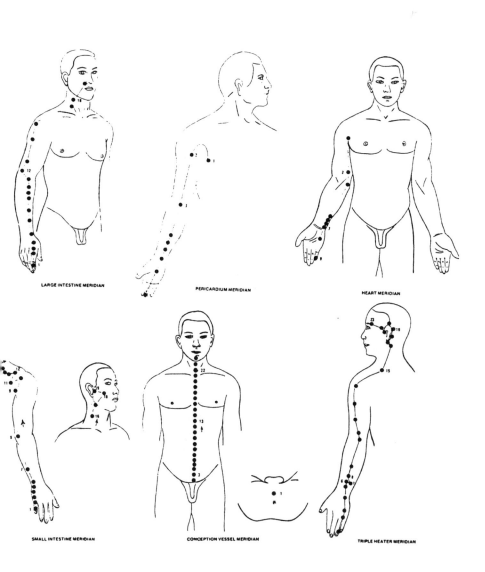

Figure 7c. Diagrams of traditional acupuncture meridians.

Today ear acupuncture has increased in use throughout the world and it is often used as a sole or supplementary treatment of some 60-70 types of ailments. In China, ear points are often stimulated in combination with body points or are used alone in acupuncture analgesia for surgery.

Currently 168 ear points have been identified, each corresponding to a different part of the body. Some of these are shown in Figure 8. The distribution of points in the ear is such that the head and neck are located in the lower portion with the remainder of the body upward.

Wen (5), of Hong Kong, used electrical stimulation of the ear for the treatment of heroin addiction. Other addictive ailments such as obesity, smoking, etc., have been so treated with small press needles, staples and beads that are inserted or sewn in place and left for varying lengths of time. The patient is instructed to press upon the bead or staple in order to self-stimulate these ear acupuncture points.

It is of interest that the ear is innervated by five major nerves. Perhaps most important of all is the fact that the concha of the ear is innervated by the vagus nerve. The concha of the ear is the only place that the vagus can be reached on the surface of the body. This may well explain its effectiveness in treating a wide variety of body ailments as well as its use in the treatment of anxiety.

MOXIBUSTION. (6) This procedures consists of the application of heat to acupuncture points. Moxa is a punk-like substance made from the herb, Artemisia Vulgaris (Mugwort). The best leaves of the plant are collected during the 5th month of the Chinese calendar, then thoroughly dried and ground to a white powder. This is mixed with tinder and formed into small cones which can be burned either directly on the skin or upon layers of soybean paste or upon small slices of ginger root. Pellets of moxa are often squeezed onto the handles of acupuncture needles and ignited. Moxa is also sold formed into sticks (cigars) which are ignited and held over the spots to be healed. This type of counterirritation formed of itself a specialty of treatment which was supposed to increase the intensity of the stimulus of acupuncture treatments at a time when electricity was not yet available. Many persons in the Orient with burn scars at acupuncture points testify to the ongoing popularity of this method of treatment. Moxibustion is simply another way of applying heat to the body.

FLUID PUNCTURE. This combines acupuncture with the injection of minute amounts of medication at acupuncture points. Local anesthetics, vitamins and hormones are often used in very minute quantities.

INCISION AND "PRICK OPEN" THERAPIES. With a heavy needle the skin is pricked open over acupuncture points and the pricking is continued into the subcutaneous fibers There should be no bleeding and the wound is treated with iodine and covered with a dressing. Incisions, 0.5 to 2 cms. long, are sometimes made in the skin over the acupuncture point. Subcutaneous, fatty

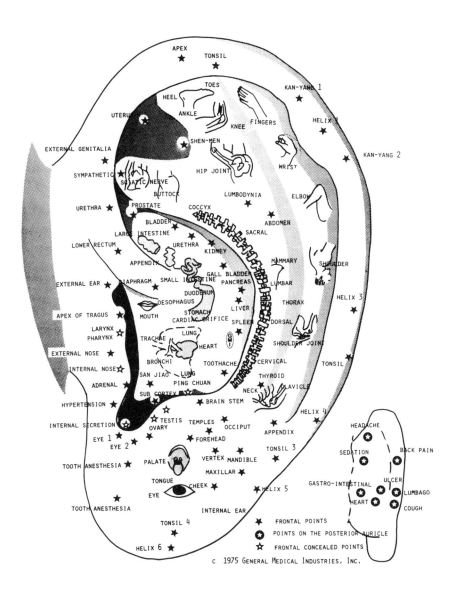

Figure 8. Theorized correspondence between designated points on the auricle and reigons of body anatomy. It is important to note that the major body organs which are innervated by the autonomic nervous system lie within the concha of the ear, an area supplied by the vagus nerve.

tissue may be removed with a hemostat and the blade of the needle pushed into the opening until a feeling of drawing, "teh chi," is experienced.

SUTURE IMPLANTATION. A piece of catgut on a round cutting needle is inserted about 1 cm from the acupuncture point and is pulled through the subcutaneous tissue in an arc pattern emerging about 1 cm. on the other side of the point. Ends of the catgut are cut close to the skin and a dressing is applied. This is left in place until eventually the suture is absorbed. The therapeutic effect is presumed to occur from the continuing irritation of the foreign body.

STAPLES. Although stainless steel staples have been commonly used at acupuncture points, these may cause infection and keloid formation. Such staples are difficult to remove without a special staple remover and, hence, patients have developed infections, as well as experienced difficulty and pain upon removal of a staple. The principle of stapling is, fortunately, on the wane.

SCALP NEEDLING. A recent method of needling was developed for the treatment of diseases of the nervous system, particularly such conditions as cerebral hemorrhage, cerebral thrombosis, Parkinson's Disease, chorea, headache and similar afflictions (7). Its basis was felt to be a reflex stimulation of the micro-circulation of the brain from needles placed in the scalp in accord with the localization of cerebro-cortical function upon the projected areas of the scalp. The needles are placed in reference to the underlying brain areas responsible for the type of function to be influenced. Particular attention was thus given to motor and sensory areas topographically located. Language areas, areas of vestibular function, areas of visceral control, etc. are similarly stimulated.

Several needles of 26-28 gauge are placed on the side contralateral to the body region to be treated. The scalp is swabbed with iodine and 2 inch long needles are inserted at an angle under the skin. After 3-5 minutes of stimulation, "teh chi" (feeling of heat, numbness, distention, soreness, etc.), has been reported in the corresponding limb or visceral area. Stimulation is given 3-4 times at a sitting with 5-10 minutes of rest intervening.

ACUPUNCTURE ANESTHESIA. In 1958 there was, in the People's Republic of China, considerable emphasis upon combining traditional Chinese medicine with Western medical science in the treatment of disease. The successful relief of post-operative pain controlled by acupuncture needling led to exploration of the use of acupuncture to replace chemical anesthetics during surgical procedures (8). Initial success with stimulation of ho ku (LI-4) , for tonsillectomy, tooth extraction and thyroidectomy led to experiments with other points and their use in a wide range of surgical procedures. Acupuncture analgesia was successfully used for many operations including major surgery of the neck, chest, limbs, and brain. It has been used in pneuomonectomy and open heart surgery. While originally as many as 80 needles were required, now adequate pain control is accomplished with only two or three needles. Points on the ears, fingers, nose, feet and lips are commonly used.

Complete anesthesia is not accomplished, yet in receptive patients, there is sufficient analgesia so that the patient rests comfortably throughout the operation. The use of acupuncture analgesia permits the patient to be awake and cooperative when that is important, as in brain and thyroid surgery. This technique avoids the slow recovery, laryngeal irritation and other untoward side effects of chemoanesthesia. As a result, post-surgical recovery time is shortened and there is early ambulation and good post-surgical control without undue sedation.

Figures vary on the reported use of acupuncture analgesia for surgical procedures in China, but it is probably used in no more than 30% of all operations. It is necessary that the patient desires this type of analgesia and is of such a disposition as to be calm despite awareness of the pulling and tugging upon tissue that occurs during the operative procedure. Patients are given some preoperative guidance and also tested as to an adequate increase of the pain threshold.

A recent study conducted in the laboratory of Ji-Sheng Han has suggested a procedure for assisting in the selection of patients suitable for acupuncture analgesia. His findings may well explain individual variations. He found that increases in pain thresholds are highly correlated with the amount of endorphin released from the central nervous system by acupuncture. Only minute amounts of endorphin are released in the brains of a subpopulation of persons who are thus not suitable for surgery under acupuncture analgesia. Therefore a measurement of endorphin levels in CSF following a challenge of acupuncture can be a useful predictor.

In some cases it is desirable to give some pre-operative medication and to have an anesthetist stand by with backup chemo-analgesia should this become necessary. The acupuncture needles are inserted 20-30 minutes before surgery and electrical stimulation is then started and continued with varying of frequencies throughout the surgery.

Although a number of surgical procedures have been successfully performed in the U.S. using acupuncture as a sole analgesic agent it is unlikely that it will become popular in this country. Patients here are accustomed to being "put to sleep" and awakened when "it is all over." Western tradition surgeons are accustomed to a completely relaxed patient and do not care for the delay and uncertainty of a surgical procedure that may be interrupted by the change over to chemical anesthesia should that be necessary in the middle of an operation.

ACU-PRESSURE. It has long been known that rubbing or pressing on an area of pain can bring about some relief. Severe pinching to produce bruises (bat go), is a part of Vietnamese folk medicine. Finger pressure (Shiatsu), ("shi"-finger, "atsu"-pressure), has long been a recognized means for modifying neural input to relieve pain in Japanese medicine. Many of the points so used correspond to acupuncture points. Some of the most effective points for producing pain and the disabling of an opponent by means of Judo are acupuncture (motor) points where strong pressure is applied directly upon an area of sensitive nerve endings. Experiments in China on animals have shown that strong pinching of the Achilles tendon can raise the pain threshold similarly, the ho ku (LI-4) point in humans has been strongly pressed or rubbed with ice to produce analgesia prior to dental extractions.

Massage in Chinese medicine following the basic formulations of energy flow and Yin/Yang balance is described for acu-pressure therapeutics (9). Thus, points for massage are the acupuncture points along the meridian lines with deep strong massage used to "tonify" or "bring Yang" and with light gentle massage to "disperse" or "sedate" and "bring Yin."

Although it has been shown that needles placed in acupuncture points with electrical stimulation produce the strongest neural activation, it would seem that pressure or massage on acupuncture (motor) points may well have some beneficial action. A school for acupuncture massage exists in Beijing and a thorough exercise of one's acupuncture points can be obtained for a minimal charge at barber shops in the People's Republic of China.

In China, the massage of eye points is a routine procedure in schools where classes stop several times a day to allow all students to participate in this method of treatment in order to strengthen vision and to prevent later eye problems. Several workers in the U.S. have reported upon the use of acu-pressure at headache points as a useful technique for the prevention of a developing headache. Pressure at feng-che (GB-20), tai yang (EM-1) and ho ku (LI-4), in succession for two minutes on each point has proved successful in reducing the intensity of head pain in a number of our patients.

In the U.S., some non-medical acupuncturists have developed techniques for "acu-pressure" to circumvent legal prohibition against the piercing of the skin with needles. The public, having little real conception of the mechanism of acupuncture, often makes little distinction between acu-pressure, acupuncture and electro-acupuncture.

SUMMARY

It is to be expected that a treatment technique that has existed for 4,000 years would have developed many variations. We have here mentioned only a few. The greatest change of all has been the addition of electrical stimulation combined with new knowledge of the anatomy and physiology of the pain pathways and what happens with electrical stimulation of certain acupuncture points. With the rapid expansion of knowledge regarding pain mechanism and pain management, the acupuncture of the future may be as different from the present physiologically based acupuncture as it is from the metaphysically based practices of traditional acupuncturists.

REFERENCES

1. Vieth, I. : **The Yellow Emperor's Classic of Internal Medicine** Univ. Ca. Press. Berkeley, CA. PP. 260, 1949.

2. Porkert M.: **The Theoretical Foundations of Chinese Medicine; Systems of Correspondence.** MIT Press, Cambridge, Mass., 368, 1974.

3. Wu-Wei-Ping; **Chinese Acupuncture.** Translated by Phillip M. Chancellor. Health Science Press, Rustington, Sussex, England, 1959.

4. Nogier, P.F.M.: **Treatise of Auriculotherapy.** Maisonneuve, France, p. 321, 1972.

5. Wen, H.L. and Cheung, S.Y.C.: Treatment of drug addiction by acupuncture and electrical stimulation **Asia J. Med.,** 9:138-141, 1973

6. **Barefoot Doctor's Manual.** The translation of the Official Chinese Paramedical Manual, Running Press, Philadelphia, PA, pp. 942, 1977.

7. Yau, P.S.: **Scalp Needling Therapy.** Medical Health Publishing Co., Hong Kong, 1975.

8. **Acupuncture Anesthesia.** Foreign Languages Press, Peking, 1972, Peoples Republic of China.

9. Borsarello, J.: **Massages in Chinese Medicine.** Maisonneuve, France, pp. 267, 1973.

Chapter II

THE MYTH OF MERIDIAN THERAPY

The term "acupuncture" has become an umbrella for a number of treatments in addition to the ancient traditional practice of placing needles and manually twisting them in some of the several hundred so-called "acupuncture points". It also applies to placing small needles, magnets, staples or taped metal pellets in some of 168 points on the ear (auriculotherapy); burning beads of moxa (artemis vulgaris) on the handles of inserted needles, or holding "cigars" of burning moxa over acupuncture points on the skin (moxibustion); simply pressing the finger deeply on acupuncture points (acu-pressure), or applying various types of electrical stimulation to inserted needles or other types of electrodes placed on acupuncture points. All of these practices are subsumed under the "acupuncture" label.

The commonly accepted explanation for the modus operandi of such treatments can be traced back to prescientific times, over 3000 years ago, when acupuncture assumed its important role in Traditional Chinese Medicine. With no knowledge of anatomy or physiology, the explanations developed were metaphysical in nature, based upon superstition, numerology and concepts from the prevailing philosophy of Taoism. It was believed that disease resulted when two theoretical forces, Yin and Yang, were out of balance. Treatments were aimed at maintaining health and producing homeostasis by increasing (tonifying) or decreasing (sedating) the forces of body energy (chhi) which traveled about in hypothesized channels beneath the surface of the skin. These channels, termed "meridians," have no demonstrated existence but have been widely accepted as an explanation for a number of holistic type practices for which there is no acceptable scientific explanation.

Numerous cultist groups have embraced this metaphysical "meridian theory" to explain their otherwise scientifically untenable practices. Reflexologists and podotherapists believe that these mythical meridians conduct fancied energy impulses from the feet where all organs and regions of the body are supposedly represented (Fig. 9). Auriculotherapists feel that the meridians begin, end, or travel through the ear in which the body is represented as an embryo, upside down (Fig. 10). Scalp-needling therapists use points on the surface of the head. Face acupuncturists believe the meridians lie on the face; Korean hand acupunc-

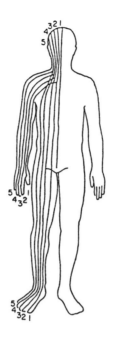

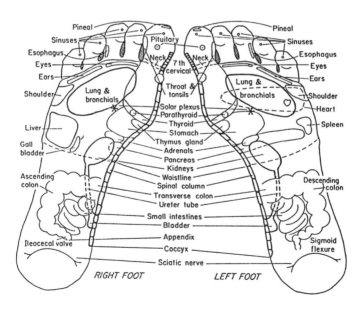

Figure 9. Foot representation of the points and meridians of Reflexology.

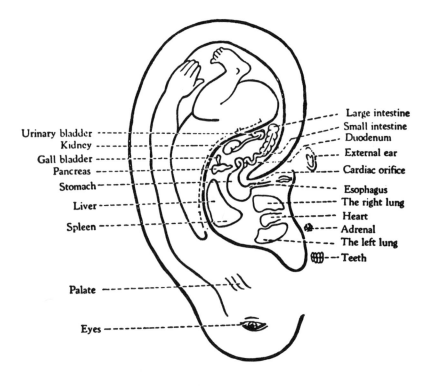

Figure 10. Corresponding anatomical representation of body areas to ear points resembling an embryo "upside down" within the auricle. From Lu, Gwei-Djen and Needham, J.: *Celestial Lancets*. Cambridge University Press, 1980, p. 427.

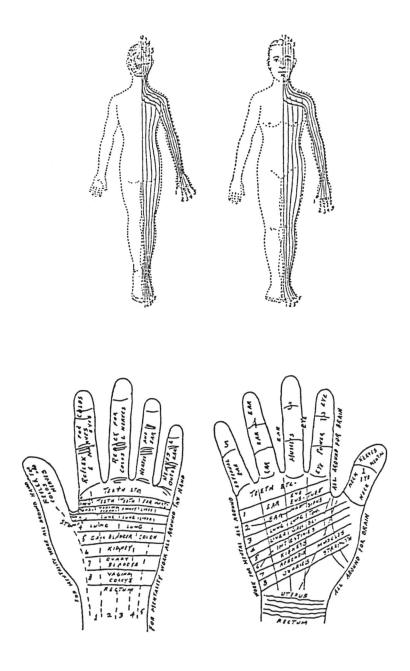

Figure 11. Hand representation of the body points and meridians of Korean Hand Acupuncture. Riley, JS, and Daglish WE: *Zone Reflex*. Mokelumne Hill, CA Health Res. 1924/42/61.

turists stimulate various organs of the body using points only on the hand (Fig. 11). For tongue acupuncturists, the tongue has its own body points, and even TENS (trans-cutaneous electrical nerve stimulation) unit salesmen show meridian charts including Chinese meridian acupuncture points for the placement of TENS electrodes!

Homeopaths, naturopaths, massage healers, laser therapists, kinesiologists, MORA color therapists, Qigong experts, magnetic therapists, practitioners of Ryodoraku and of Traditional Chinese Medicine, as well as chiropractors practicing sacral apex adjustments, use the meridian concept to explain their various manipulations upon the body. Great claims are made for all these therapies. With "cure-all" treatments, and particularly those that carry the added charisma of the mysterious Orient, a strong 30 percent placebo rate of success occurs.

Upon this placebo based reputation the meridian therapies have flourished over the years. All books and lectures on acupuncture and related subjects simply repeat, in various elaborate forms, the ancient myth of meridian therapy. Such lack of a proven scientific basis for these procedures has been no hindrance to the practice of acupuncture by both medically trained and various non-medical persons.

From the foregoing it might appear that any physician with scientific medical training would be justified in completely rejecting acupuncture as a practice unworthy of serious attention. To do so however might well lead to the neglect of an important avenue for patient care, for acupuncture has been shown to be an effective therapy.

Concurrently, with the growth of cultic acupuncture, there has also been a great surge of scientific interest and knowledge about the neurophysiology of pain. Along with Melzac and Wall's introduction of the gate theory (1), there came increased knowledge of the role of polypeptides in brain function, the widespread use of TENS units and an explosion of data about the neural pathways involved in pain.

Research on the mechanism of acupuncture analgesia, especially the seminal findings of Han and his co-workers at the Medical University of Beijing (2), has now placed Traditional Chinese Acupuncture in proper perspective. No longer can any scientifically trained physician seriously accept metaphysical meridian theory as an explanation for electro-acupuncture. Rather, we must now view the metaphysics of traditional acupuncture as an important antecedent development in the history of medicine - one stone in the foundation of the specialty of algology. For it is upon these formulations, developed in pre-scientific times, that Han and others have been able to construct a series of experiments that have resulted in a scientifically tenable explanation of how electrical stimulation can activate the body's own pain modulation mechanisms.

Han has shown that by changing the frequency of stimulation, without altering the needle insertion or electrode placement, different brain neuropeptides concerned with anti-nociceptive processes can be activated (3). Thus it becomes clear that acupuncture is not **point specific**, but rather it is **frequency specific**.

We can now discard the ancient charts of points placed on meridian channels. Early work from our laboratories (4), supported by findings from Liu (5), Gunn (6,7) and others, demonstrated that the most important acupuncture points are simply the points used by electromyographers. Only a few of these points are required for effective treatment of pain. Ho ku (motor point of the adductor pollicus and interosseus muscle between thumb and forefinger), is useful for pain problems in the upper half of the body, Tsu san li (motor point of the tibialis anticus), can be used for the lower half of the body. Either of these points can significantly raise the pain threshold. By stimulation of such points, Han has demonstrated a rise in the level of endorphins and dynorphins as shown by monitoring the spinal fluid of human volunteers (8).

Thus the fact that meridians do not exist, in no way nullifies the value of acupuncture treatments. As Felix Mann once said "Traditional acupuncturists get good results but for the wrong reasons". (9)

Similarly, one need not accept the elaborate theories of auriculotherapy to explain the mechanism of needles inserted in the ear. In no place does a study of human biology or comparative anatomy give any reason to believe that small patches of skin on the surface of the body are specific key points which act as control centers for modifying functions of body organs and parts. It makes no more sense for the ear than it does for the foot, the hand or the tongue, each of which has their proponents for such mystical explanatory theories.

In the 1960's, Wen of Hong Kong found that a needle in the concha of the ear, when stimulated electrically, was useful in treating heroin addicts (10). Since then a number of workers have supported and extended his original observations. Recently some have, following the elaborate theories of Nogier (11), stated that needles placed at points in the ear labeled as "lung," "liver," "sympathetic," etc., have specific demonstrable physiological actions and can produce results without the necessity for electrical stimulation. It is of more than passing interest that these useful points are all located in the concha of the ear. One study (12), used such conchal points as "active" points and non-conchal points for "control" points in patients being treated for cocaine dependence. This study showed positive results, thus indicating that the concha is an active region. It is known that this area is innervated by the vagus nerve and hence the most acceptable explanation is not one of many individual mystical points located "as on an embryo upside down", but rather, that the concha as a whole is the active vagal area (13). A single electrode placed anywhere in the concha, with electrical stimulation as used by Wen, would seem the most reasonable way to produce results from ear stimulation. As for the theories of auriculotherapy, is it not more likely that human beings would devise metaphysical explanations for the results of their treatments than that nature would go out of her way to create an area of the body deviating from all known and usual biological principles?

It would appear that such acceptance of the mystical, as opposed to the scientific, is typical of what occurs among persons who embrace and practice various ancient healing cults. For example, increasingly at conventions and seminars on traditional Chinese medicine and acupuncture, the so called Qigong masters have been making an appearance. Books, lectures and videotapes on Qigong methodology have found a ready market in the U.S. Qigong is a part of ancient traditional Chinese medicine. It is divided into two parts internal Qigong and external Qigong. Some say the former is scientific in the sense that it is primarily a deep breathing exercise that could be beneficial to health, relaxation, concentration, etc. External Qigong functions as a paranormal event. Proponents state that: "It can enable you to emit powerful forces from touching them," and "can cause healing and various chemical reactions to occur at great distances from the Qigong expert." It works, however, only if you "are not skeptical." Lin Zixin (14), former editor of China's *Science and Technology Daily,* invited an American delegation from the **Committee for Scientific Investigation of Claims of the Paranormal** to China to test the powers of Qigong. The results of their investigations, that proved these powers fraudulent, have been published in the *Skeptical Inquiror* and recorded on videotape. (15).

Thus it is time to discard the ancient metaphysical theories that were formerly the only existing explanations for the action of acupuncture. We now know not only that acupuncture works but also how it works. Modern scientific techniques have been able to "separate the wheat from the chaff". There are good acceptable scientific explanations for those parts of Traditional Chinese Medicine that are useful therapeutic additions to the armamentarium of modern practicing physicians. As for the myth of meridian therapy, mysterious theories of auriculotherapy, Qigong and the like, they should all be looked upon as interesting anecdotes from the distant past.

REFERENCES

1. Melzac, R., and Wall, P.: Pain Mechanism; a New Theory. *Science* 1965. 150:971-973.

2. Han, JS.: *The neurochemical basis of pain relief by acupuncture. A collection of papers, 1973-1987.* Beijing Medical University, Beijing, China, 1987.

3. Han, JS.: and Sun SL: Differential release of Encephalon and Dynorphin by Low and High Frequency Electroacupuncture in the Central Nervous System (Part I). *Acupuncture: the Scientific International Journal.* 1:19-027, 1990.

4. Brown, ML, Ulett GA, Stern JA.: Acupuncture loci: Techniques for location. *Am J Chin Med* 1974: 2(1): 57-74

5. Liu KY, Varela M. Oswald R.: The correspondence between some motor points and acupuncture loci. **Am J. Chin Med** 1975; 3:347-358

6. Gunn, CC.: Motor Points and Motor Lines, *Am. J. Acupuncture* 6:55-58, 1978

7. Gunn, CC.: Type IV Acupuncture Points *Am.J. Acupuncture* 5:51-52, 1977.

8. Han, JS: (Talk given at the Missouri Institute of Mental Health, Aug. 1991).

9. Mann, Felix: Personal communication.

10. Wen, H., Cheung S.: Treatment of drug addition by acupuncture and electrical stimulation, **Asian Journal of Medicine** 1973, 9:138-141.

11. Nogier, PFM: **Treatise of Auriculotherapy** Maisonneuve, France, 1972.

12. Lipton, DS, Brewington, V., Smith MO: Paper presented at the NIDA Technical Review Meeting, Advances in Cocaine Treatment, Bethesda, Maryland Aug 16, 1990.

13. Ulett, GA: **Principles and Practice of Physiologic Acupuncture.** Warren Green, St. Louis 1982.

14. **Skeptical Briefs.** 1 (3) August 1991.

15. Kurtz, P., Alcock, J., Frazier, K., Karr, B., Klass, PJ. and Randi, J.: Testing Psi Claims in China: Visit of CSICOP Delegation. **Skeptical Inquirer,** 12 (4): 364-375, 1988.

Chapter III

BRIDGING THE GAP FROM TRADITIONAL TO PHYSIOLOGIC ACUPUNCTURE

Acupuncture has existed in China for over 4,000 years. It spread to Korea in approximately 300 A.D. and on to Japan in the 17th century. By the year 1800 there was considerable interest in Europe where acupuncture remains a commonly used therapy. The World Health Organization estimates that acupuncture is now a major mode of treatment for one third of the world's population.

Acupuncture was but little known in the United States until relatively recent years. It was mentioned in a surgical treatise by Billroth in 1863, and again by Sir William Osler in 1912 (1). In that edition of his book **Principles and Practice of Medicine**, he stated, "For lumbago, acupuncture is, in acute cases, the most efficient treatment." This statement was deleted from subsequent editions. There was then a hiatus of some 60 years before this advice was again taken seriously by physicians in the United States.

Increased attention to acupuncture began at the time of the visit of President Nixon to China in 1971. At that time a member of the press corps, James Reston, had an emergency appendectomy performed in China. On his return to the United States he reported upon his relief from post-appendectomy pain by means of acupuncture. With parting of the "bamboo curtain," there was considerable interest in things Chinese and the idea that tiny needles could relieve pain fascinated the American public. Its use as an anesthetic in surgical procedures created interest among members of the medical profession. Reports in the popular press presented acupuncture as a "cure-all." This created an instant demand for such treatment by patients with chronic pain and other complaints of varied etiology.

Explanation of the acupuncture phenomenon in terms of Yin/Yang and other Oriental metaphysical and superstitious ideas was unacceptable to Americans who described its action as hypnosis, placebo or simply Oriental stoicism. In 1972, The American Medical Association cautioned against acupuncture quackery and since then has labeled acupuncture as an "experimental procedure." (2)

The public, however, was not to be put off. Patients with chronic pain sought this treatment with great hope and rising to meet their desire were hundreds of persons with no formal medical training. Such practitioners immersed themselves in the theories of ancient Chinese metaphysical methods of diagnosis and treatment despite the fact that these had no basis in modern medical science. The number of such practitioners increased to thousands and was joined by chiropractors, naturopaths, homeopaths, and some M.D.'s and D.O.'s who were comfortable in ignoring the advances of modern medical science and regressing to an acceptance of metaphysical theories of disease dating from prescientific times.

Some of these groups organized and exerted pressure upon state legislatures for recognition. As a result, as of this writing, 22 states have passed regulations certifying or licensing persons for the practice of acupuncture. In twelve states, persons with no medical training are certified as primary health care practitioners (3). In California, applicants for such certification are not even required to know the English language because examinations can be taken in Chinese. As a result of this confusion, and because available books and courses are simply repetitions of ancient philosophical concepts, scientifically oriented American physicians have been most reluctant to add this treatment method to their clinical practice, thus depriving their patients of what has proven be a valuable and effective treatment.

Two leading hypnotists with vast experience in hypnosis (4, 5), but little with acupuncture, stated early on that acupuncture was a kind of Oriental hypnotic induction ceremony. As familiarity with acupuncture increased such opinions changed. Thus Patrick Wall stated in 1972, "My own belief is that...acupuncture is an effective use of hypnosis." (6) In 1974, after a study tour of China, he retracted that statement. (7). Ronald Katz stated, "I have assisted at four operations under acupuncture anesthesia and many more than that under hypnosis. The patients behave differently. Those under hypnosis are...seemingly unaware of what is going on around them. Patients under acupuncture were part of the team, joking laughing and commenting freely." (8) My coworkers and I received the first grant given by NIH for the study of acupuncture. Our investigation compared the use of acupuncture and hypnosis for the treatment of experimentally induced pain. As our poor hypnotic subjects did just as well as the good hypnotic subjects, it was our conclusion that acupuncture is not hypnosis. (9)

In this research project we also found that some of the designated traditional acupuncture points had a standing electrical potential different from surrounding skin.(10) Our work was done with a roving electrode that exerted no pressure upon the skin. This was necessary as we found that so called "point finders" that measured skin resistance gave false measurements which could be altered by simply changing the amount of pressure upon the skin. It has been our interpretation that these standing electrical potentials were produced by changes in the underlying anatomy, namely so called neuro-vascular hilae. These are areas where the major innervation of a muscle occurs and where the penetrating nerves are accompanied by entering blood vessels. Our belief in this regard has been supported by observations of Liu et al. (11) They had "blinded" acupuncturists identify major acupuncture points and compared these to the findings of "blinded" electromyographers who identified the points used in electromyography. Many of the more commonly used acupuncture points were found to be identical with EMG points. Other points, not identical, were very close. This was not unexpected. At a meeting in Beijing that I attended, a group of experienced acupuncturists agreed that among them there were significant variations in their location of points. In an attempt to minimize such variations the Chinese used the "cun" or body inch to measure distances from recognizable anatomical landmarks as they counted various acupuncture points. This measure was the distance between two folds of the middle phalanx of the patient's middle finger in bent position. Although not entirely accurate, it usually did vary in a direction corresponding to the size of the individual.

Gunn (12) speaks of the importance not only of motor points (points used in electromyography, neuro-vascular hilae) but also points on Golgi tendon organs and of Travell's trigger points (13), which coincide with the "ah shi" points of acupuncture described by Chung (14). These are points that the patient designates by responding to the examiners probing finger saying "oh yes" or in Chinese "ah shi."

Our studies also delineated the importance of using progressively stronger stimuli in order to elicit the most beneficial results in the control of experimental pain (Fig. 13). We studied the results of needles under four conditions: (1) placed in false or "placebo" points without stimulation, (2) placed in false points with electrical stimulation, (3) placed in true points without electrical stimulation, and (4) placed in true points with electrical stimulation. The relief from needles in true (motor) points with electrical stimulation gave the greatest relief from the experimentally produced ischemic pain or the pain of electric shock. This relief was as great as that produced by the injection intramuscularly of 10 mg of morphine sulfate given 20 minutes prior to testing.(15)

This use of electrical stimulation of acupuncture needles is not a recent phenomenon. It is reported that Gennai Hiraga of Envo, Japan used electro-acupuncture in 1764. In 1825, Chevalier Sarlandiere of France described the application of an electric current from Leyden jars applied to inserted acupuncture needles. In 1973, Wen, of Hong Kong used electrical stimulation of the ear for the successful treatment of heroin addiction.(16) Papers by Laitinen (17) and Fox and Melzack (18), have compared acupuncture (needles twirled), without electrical stimulation and stimulation done with electrically stimulated conductive polymer electrodes (TENS), for the treatment of low-back pain. They found that in general acupuncture and TENS treatments were equally effective. In view

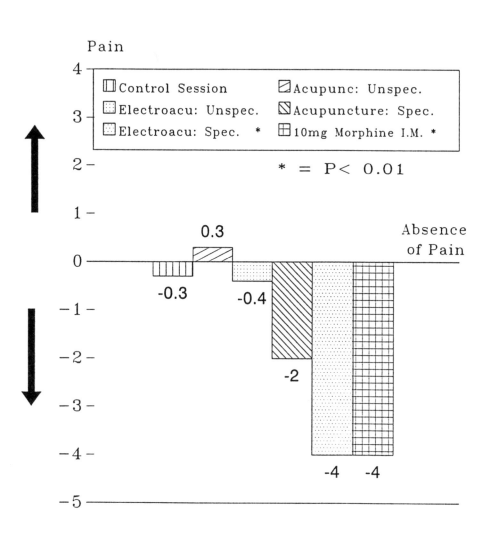

Figure 13. Changes in Subjective Experience with Different Pain Challengers to Experimental Pain (N:20)

of the fact that electrical stimulation has been found to increase the effectiveness of acupuncture needles, a study of TENS and electroacupuncture would have added important information to these studies. Today in all countries of the world, modern acupuncturists have found the application of electricity to needles and other electrodes a most effective way to enhance treatment procedures.

Coincidently with the greater use of traditional acupuncture treatments by non-medical groups, there has also been a gradual increase of interest by physicians. Concurrently there has been, in this decade of the brain, a great leap forward in our understanding of pain mechanisms and acupuncture. In fact it can now truly be said that the meridians are a myth, that acupuncture points may well be motor points, that auriculotherapy is primarily a stimulation of the vagus nerve, and as will be explained further, acupuncture analgesia is less point specific than it is frequency specific.

REFERENCES

1. Osler, Wm. **Principles and Practice of Medicine** 8th Ed. D. Appleton and Col. N.Y. 1912.

2. AMA Council on Scientific Affairs: **Reports of the Council on Scientific Affairs of the American Medical Association 1981.** Chicago, American Medical Association, 1982

3. Training and Certification of Acupuncturists. **The American Acupuncturist** Official Publication of the AAAOM. X: Summer, 1991, p. 11.

4. Spiegel, H. and Spiegel, D.: **Trance and Treatment** Basic Books, N.Y. pp 370, 19788.

5. Kroger, WS, D.: *Hypnotism and Acupuncture.* JAMA. 2201012, 1972.

6. Wall, P.: An Eye on the Needle. **New Scientist,** 55:129-131, 1972.

7. Wall, P.: Acupuncture Revisited. **New Scientist.** 4:31-34, 1974.

8. Katz, RL, Kao, CY, Spiegel, H., and Katz, OT.: Acupuncture Hypnosis. **Advances in Neurology.** 4:819-825, 1974.

9. Parwatikar, S., Brown, M., Stern, J., Ulett, GA. and Sletten, IW. :Acupuncture, Hypnosis and Experimental Pain I. Study with Volunteers. Acup **and Electrotherap. Res.** 3:161-190, 1978.

10. Brown, ML, Ulett, GA, and Stern, JA.: Acupuncture Loci: Techniques for Location. **Amer. J. Chinese Med.** 3(1) 67-74, 1974.

11. Liu, YK, Varela, M and Oswald, R.,: The Correspondence between Some Motor Points and Acupuncture Loci. **Amer. J. Chin. Med.** 3:347-358, 1975.

12. Gunn, CC.: Type IV Acupuncture Points, **Am. J. Acupuncture** 5:51-58.

13. Travell, J.: Referred Pain from Skeletal Muscle. **New York State J. Med.** 55: 331-

14. Chung, C.: **Ah-Shih Point, The Pressure Pain Point in Acupuncture.** Chen Kwan Book Co. Ltd. Taipei, Taiwan, P. 212, 1982

15. Saletu, B., Saletu, M., Stern, JA., Ulett, GA., and Sletten IW.: Hypno-Analgesia and Acupuncture Analgesia: A Neurophysiologic reality? **Neuropsychobiology,** 1:218-242, 1975

16. Wen, HC., and Teo, SW: Experience in the treatment of Drug Addiction by electro-Acupuncture. **Mod. Med. Asia.** 11:23-24, 1975.

17. Laitinen, J.: Acupuncture and transcutaneous electric Stimulation in the Treatment of Chronic Sacrolumbalgia and Ischialgia. **Amer. J. Chinese Medicine** 4 (2):1689-175, 1976.

18. Fox, EJ., Melzack, R.,: Transcutaneous Electrical Stimulation and Acupuncture: Comparison of treatment for Low-Back Pain. **Pain.** 2:141-148, 1976.

Chapter IV

SCIENTIFIC STUDIES AND THEORIES OF ACUPUNCTURE ACTION

NEUROCHEMICAL MECHANISMS OF ACUPUNCTURE

Systematic studies on the neurochemical mechanisms of acupuncture have been conducted by Dr. Ji-Sheng Han and his associates at Beijing University.(1) This outstanding work has not only removed the veil of metaphysics from the over 3,000-year-old Chinese medical treatment, but has vastly advanced knowledge of the brain's circuitry concerned with pain perception and its modulation.

Initially, human volunteers in Dr. Han's laboratory, were given electro-acupuncture and their pain thresholds were measured over time. The analgesic effect gradually increased, peaked, and then gradually declined. Although the intensity of this effect varied among individuals, it could be elicited from different points on the body and had approximately the same half life. These observations confirmed the analgesic action of acupuncture and caused Han to believe that some chemical substance was responsible for acupuncture analgesia. This conclusion prompted the use of the technique of cross-infusion of cerebrospinal fluid between two rabbits only one of which received electro-acupuncture. Following the electro-acupuncture, the cerebrospinal perfusate of one rabbit was then injected into the cerebral ventricle of the rabbit which did not receive acupuncture. Surprisingly the pain threshold of both rabbits increased, suggesting that the analgesic action of acupuncture is mediated by substances produced or released in the brain. These substances with their analgesic property had been transferred from one animal to the other.(2)

Encouraged by the new techniques of neurobioassay (3), Han then embarked upon a series of experiments aimed at discovering which neurohumors were responsible for this transfer of analgesic properties. Early studies (4), showed that one of the classical neurotransmitters, serotonin, was important for mediating acupuncture analgesia. It was found that the effect of acupuncture analgesia was markedly decreased when the brain was depleted of 5-hydroxytryptophan (5-HTP), the serotonin precursor.(4) Similarly, chlorimipramine, a tricyclic compound that selectively facilitated serotonergic transmission, potentiated the effect of acupuncture analgesia.(5)

Enhancement of the action of the endorphin system, and thus, enhancement of acupuncture analgesia, may be induced by D-amino acids (6), such as D-phenylalanine (7). The role of midbrain monoamines is of importance. Parachlorphenylanine (PCTA), which blocks the bio-synthesis of serotonin blocks acupuncture analgesia in the rabbit.(8) Methysergide, which blocks serotonin receptors, has been shown to have a similar effect in mice.(9) Han, *et al*, (10), showed that forebrain serotonin is more important than spinal cord serotonin for acupuncture analgesia. Yohimbine, a norepinephrine alpha-antagonist, given systemically, blocks acupuncture analgesia.(11) The central catecholamine, norepinephrines, was found to have an antagonistic effect upon acupuncture in the brain (10), but was essential for the mediation of acupuncture analgesia in the spinal cord. Hammond (12), combined intrathecal antagonists (methysergide for serotonin and phenotolamine for norephinephrine) and produced marked antagonism of descending analgesia from brainstem stimulation. Thus, there is good collective evidence that the monoamines, serotonin and norepinephrine, play a role in acupuncture analgesia.

In the 1950s, Chang (13), discovered that the site of analgesic action of morphine is in the brain. Knowledge of nature's own morphine-like substance, the endorphins, opened up a whole new chapter in pain research. There is much evidence to support the role of endorphins in acupuncture analgesia. Mayer, *et al*, (14), studied laboratory-induced tooth pain in humans, producing acupuncture analgesia by manual twirling of needles in LI-4 the first dorsal interosseus motor point of the hand. In a double blind study they found that naloxone blocked this analgesia while saline did not.

Microinjection studies of naloxone into the periacqueductal gray or intrathecally over the spinal cord decreased acupuncture analgesia in rats and rabbits.(15) Other sites that do not contain endorphins show no such naloxone effects. It was found that opioid peptides could be grouped into the enkephalins, endorphins, and dynorphins. Working with Terenius, Han (16), using the antibody microinjection technique, showed that enkephalins were mediators for acupuncture analgesia in both the brain and spinal cord, whereas Beta-endorphin was effective in the brain but not in the spinal cord. In a carefully conducted experiment Han and Xie (17), also showed that dynorphin antiserum blocked acupuncture analgesia in rabbits. Figure 13 illustrates Han's work using antibodies as a tool for analyzing the action of opioid peptides.

It was found that dynorphins (18), were effective in the spinal cord but not in the brain. Thus, in summary, it could be seen that acupuncture could release B-endorphins and enkephalins in the brain and dynorphins and enkephalins in the spinal cord.

Peetz and Pomeranz (19), bred a strain of mice with a congenital deficiency in endorphin receptors. These mice produced less than half the electro-acupuncture analgesia seen in normal strains of mice. These workers hypothesized that the 30% of humans who do not respond to acupuncture analgesia may well have a genetic deficiency in opiate receptors in the central nervous system.

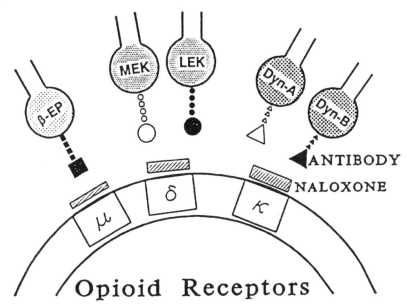

Figure 13. Antibody as a specific tool to analyze different kinds of opioid peptides in mediating acupuncture analgesia. B-EP=Beta endorphin, MEK=Methionin-enkephalin, LEK=Leucin-enkephalin, Dyn-A=dynorphin A, Dyn-B=dynorphin B. (Han , JS in Press.)

Important correlates of the endorphin acupuncture analgesis hypothesis are found in the reports by Sjolund, *et al* (20), that endorphins are increased in cerebrospinal fluid with acupuncture stimulation. A doubling of the endorphin level in cerebrospinal fluid occurred within 30 minutes of stimulation. Similarly, an increase of 50% in blood cortisol occurred with stimulation at acupuncture points but there was no such increase with stimulation at non-acupuncture points.(21)

Traditional acupuncturists have observed that different types of needle manipulation at the same point could bring about different results. Needling at ST-36 (anterior tibialis motor point) could, for example, treat diarrhea in one case and constipation in another. A possible explanation of the mechanism involved was found when it was shown that low-frequency (2-4 Hz) stimulation could cause preferentially a release of met-enkephalin whereas high-frequency (80-100 Hz) stimulation would selectively release dynorphins.(22) Pomeranz and Cheng (23), showed that naloxone would block low frequency (4 Hz) electroacupuncture. Acupuncture analgesia produced by low-frequency stimulation is endorphinergic (24, 25). Acupuncture analgesia produced by high-frequency stimulation is not affected by naloxone, but is monoaminergic and can be enhanced by the serotonin precursor 5-HTP. (10)

It was shown by Pomeranz (26), and Watkins and Mayer (27), that antagonists such as naloxone work best when given before the acupuncture treatment and may fail to reverse the acupuncture analgesia once it is established. This may be due to the fact that naloxone binds poorly to kappa receptors, and, hence, may have difficulty overcoming the effect of dynorphin. Since the analgesic effect of metenkephalin is mediated mainly by mu and delta receptors and that of dynorphins by kappa receptors, it becomes apparent that by using specific parameters of electrical stimulation of acupuncture needles one might be able to switch on and off the activity of various peptidergic systems of the central nervous system for different therapeutic purposes. Figure 14a, illustrates the neural pathways that mediate analgesia with stimulation by electro-acupuncture or TENS and b, the synergistic effect on analgesia of opioid peptides so

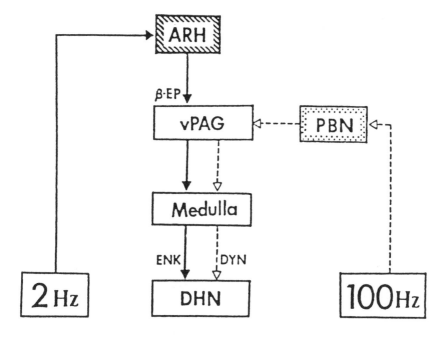

Figure 14a. Neural pathways mediating analgesia induced by electro-acupuncture or TENS of different frequencies. ARH: acrcuate nucelus of hypothalamus, vPAG: ventral PAG, PBN: parabrachial nucleus, HN: dorsal horn neurone. (Han, JS. In press)

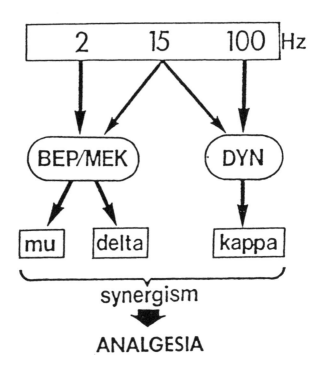

Figure 14b. Electroacupuncture or TENS at different frequencies may release different kinds of opioid peptides in CNS, acting on different types of opioid receptor to produce analgesia. (Han JS. in press)

released.

The work of Han has clearly shown that it is the frequency rather than the intensity of the stimulation that is of the utmost importance in producing acupuncture analgesia (28), and thus it may be that lack of response to electro-acupuncture could well be overcome by finding the proper parameters of stimulation for each individual.

Because the acupuncture effect depends upon manipulation of biochemical systems that have widespread effects throughout the central nervous system it has become apparent that the effectiveness of acupuncture stimulation is not dependent upon the specific placement of needles. It is only important perhaps that some locations have a greater overall effect than others. Thus, a needle placed in ho ku (dorsal interosseus motor point of the thumb) or any other motor point located distally on the upper extremity, may produce widespread analgesic effects through actuating the Beta-endorphinergic and enkephalinergic system. Simultaneous stimulation of another point, for example, tsu san li on the leg (tibialis anterior motor point), might produce an additive effect. On the other hand, if one wishes to stimulate the release of dynorphins for local effect mediated by spinal cord nerves, stimulation of motor points in the neurotome supplying the area of pain could conceivably add yet another dimension of analgesia.

Han also demonstrated the importance of the phenomenon of acupuncture tolerance.(29) With continuous stimulation, the acupuncture analgesia may completely disappear within 6 hours. It appears that angiotensin and cholecystokinin-8 may be important in antagonizing acupuncture analgesia. The implication here is that electro-acupuncture stimulation should be given intermittently. Therefore, clinically, electro-acupuncture stimulation is often given for periods of 20-30 minutes daily with a stimulus that delivers alternating low (2-4 Hz) and high (80-100 Hz) frequencies.

In 1965, Melzack and Wall (30) proposed the gate theory as a mechanism for understanding the modulation of pain (Figure 15). In the years that have followed, our understanding of the mechanism by which pain can be modulated has greatly increased. Han's more complex diagram (Figure 16), clearly delineates anatomic areas that are important way-stations in the central nervous system network responsible for mediation and control for noxious input.(31) Four nuclei; accumbens, amygdala, habenual, and the preriacqueductal gray, were found to be sensitive areas where naloxone was most effective in blocking acupuncture analgesia. It became clear that there was a mesolimbic loop (32), with connections between accumbens, habenula, and periacqueductal gray, and if this loop was broken at any of the nuclei the impulses necessary for the modulation of pain at the dorsal horn neurone of the spinal cord would be interrupted.

It was also found that the hindbrain neural circuits are essential for control of the spinal gating mechanisms. If the upward flow from acupuncture stimulation is blocked supratentorially, there is considerable interference with the analgesic effect.(32)

The role of the hypothalamus is clearly indicated. All of the Beta-endorphin containing cells of the brain are found in the arcuate nucleus of the hypothalamus and in the pituitary gland.(33) From the arcuate nucleus Beta-endorphins are released that stimulate long reaching axones to affect midbrain pain control mechanisms.(34) Lesions in the arcuate nucleus can abolish acupuncture analgesia in a rat.(35)

Brain and blood levels of Beta-endorphin are elevated by stress.(36) Although we are concerned mainly with the effect of acupuncture on pain in this discussion, it is important to note that other effects of acupuncture, such as upon infections and the immune system, may be attributed to the fact that the precursor molecule for Beta-endorphin is the same precursor molecule from which adrenocorticotropic hormone is produced. Thus when a molecule of endorphin is produced by electro-acupuncture stimulation, a molecule of ACTH is simultaneously released.

In summary, acupuncture stimulates the endogenous pain-modulating system to release serotonin, opioid substances, and other transmitters at three levels of the central nervous system, the spinal cord, the thalamus, and the cerebral cortex, thus serving to dampen the perception and transmission of nociceptive signals. How these impulses enter the central nervous system to produce the neurochemical effects demonstrated above is, of course, of the utmost importance to an understanding of the acupuncture phenomenon.

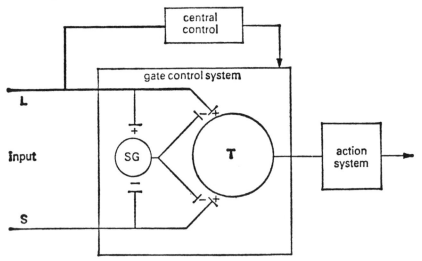

Figure 15. Schematic diagram of the gate-control theory of pain mechanisms. From Melzack, R., and Wall, P.: Pain mechanisms: A new theory. *Science*, 150:971-73, 1965. Copyright 1965 , by the American Association for the Advancement of Science.

PERCEPTION AND TRANSMISSION OF PAIN SIGNALS The mechanism of electro-acupuncture pain control through neurotransmitter release has been conclusively demonstrated and its superiority over simply needling without electric stimulation is generally recognized. As we have pointed out, needles alone have a strong placebo effect. Whether, in addition, the penetration of a needle into muscle fiber may also produce some local physiological effect that has a bearing on pain modulation has been a subject of considerable speculation. Peng and Greenfield have reviewed this matter (37), and listed some of the possible mechanisms that might be important. Among them they mention: a current of injury in the neighborhood of 3-6 nano-amperes that is equivalent to the optimal current for tissue-regeneration, axon reflex release of histamine, and stimulation of the nerve endings of the calcitonin-gene related-peptide (CGRP) containing primary afferent nerves. These release acetylcholine which produces dilation of blood vessels in the spastic ischemic muscle. They point out that the effect of a single needle penetration, due to such mechanisms can be both immediate and long lasting.

Melzack and Melinkoff (38), raised the pain threshold by stimulating the cat's midbrain reticular formation. Andersson concluded that stimulation of the muscle afferents at intensities activating high-threshold nerves can produces acupuncture effects.(39) A sensation of "Teh Chi" (swelling, drawing, soreness and numbness), that is said to be essential for obtaining therapeutic effectiveness of acupuncture, arises from A-delta fibers and, thus, is mainly derived from muscle nerves. As noted, injections of novocaine into the skin does not block the acupuncture effect whereas deep injection into the muscle tissue often does.

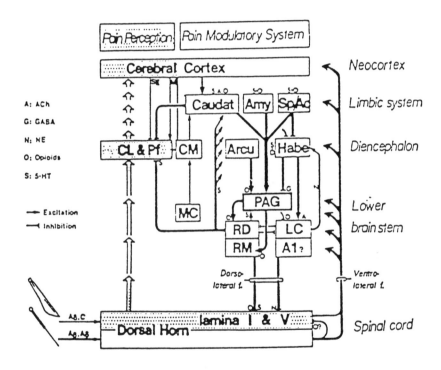

Figure 16. Diagram showing the possible mechanisms of acupuncture analgesia. A1= perikarya of noradrenergic-neurons with descending fibers to the spinal cord (Whether it is group A1, or A5-7 remains toe be identifeid); Ac=nucleus accumbens; Amy=nucleus amygdala; Arcu=nucleus arcuatus hypothalami; Caudat=nucelus caudatus; CL=nucleu centrolateralis hypothalami; CM=nucleus centroemedianus hypothalami; Habe=nucelus habenula; LC=locus ceruleus; MC=nucleus megalocellularis; PAG=periaqueductal grey; Pf=nucleus parafascicularis; RD=nucleus raphe dorsalis; RM=nucleus raphe magnus; Sp=septum

Once pain signals have entered the dorsal horn of the spinal cord they spread widely throughout the central nervous system. Andersson and co-workers in Göteborg (40,41,42,43) working with pain from tooth pulp stimulation in the cat, ascertained that information interpreted as pain reached the cortex by multiple paths, some proceeding directly over the thalamocortical pathways and ultimately terminating in laminae IV of the cortex. Studies from China (44), showed that the stimulated potentials in the sensory cortex could be abolished by stimulation of the acupuncture point LI-4 (motor point of the dorsal interosseus muscle).

The widespread nature of pain responses has also been confirmed by observations of an increased cerebral blood flow over large regions of the cerebral cortex after a noxious stimulus.(45) This has also been beautifully demonstrated by the work of Hand (46), who indexed pain pathways throughout the central nervous system by means of labeled deoxyglucose. He then studied the powerful acupuncture point tsu san li (anterior tibialis motor point), and detected a statistically significant decrease in neuronal activity at representative points throughout the central nervous system pain network when acupuncture was delivered simultaneously with the pain stimulus. Taken together, such explanations clearly demonstrated the effect of acupuncture as an electrophysiologic event modifying pain impulses.

While such explanations may serve to describe the modulation of acute, ongoing pain phenomena, they still leave questions regarding the perception and control of chronic pain. When acupuncture is used as an analgesic for surgery, stimulation is started 20-40 minutes prior to the operation to permit a build-up (recruiting, deepening) of sufficient analgesia to allow surgery with sensation but without pain. When the analgesia-producing electro-acupuncture stimulation is stopped, it has been observed that while diminishing, the effect lasts over a period of 30 minutes or more. What, then, might be the mechanism for relief from chronic pain over even longer periods of time or permanently?

It seems probable on the basis of known physiology that in establishing conditions of chronic pain, the ancient, slowly conducting system of C fibers takes dominion over the more phylogenetically recent, rapidly conducting large myelinated fibers. With continuing stimulation from tissue damage or irritation, the pain becomes continuous or chronically intermittent. Such continuous bombardment of the neuraxis by noxious stimuli could well produce a kindling effect (47) within neurone pools of the central nervous system such that reverberating circuits are created with self-perpetuation or continuation of the pain sensation. This type of self-sustaining activity (Figure 17) was described by Lorente de No (48), and Dusser de Barenne and McCulloch (49). Such circuits at the spinal cord level have been described by Loesser *et al* in the deafferented spinal cord in a patient with continuing paraplegic pain.(50) This self-generated abnormal bursting activity in the spinal cord has also been described by the above workers in the cat with chronic deafferentation. Such spinal reverberating circuits could serve to constantly activate pathways. This might explain the continuing memory of pain in the central nervous system long after the original tissue injury has been repaired. In the case of phantom limb pain it would appear that the activity continues to reverberate in the central circuits previously utilized by the now nonexistent limb.

An alternative mechanism could be a malfunction of the system for production and control of brain hormones that relate to the pain experience. Thus, the noxious impulses could well produce a dysregulation of those homeostatic mechanisms that are normally responsible for a return to the resting stage after the sensation of acute pain has given a warning for the location and extent of tissue damage. A continuing very intense pain stimulus could presumably result in either an excessive production of the peptides responsible for the transmission of pain impulses or a breakdown in the function of those structures responsible for the production of enkephalins necessary for suppression of neuronal activity in the pain pathways.

Another possible scenario occurs when the pain impulse spreads to involve the intermediolateral cell column (Figure 18) of the spinal cord and the sympathetic nervous system neurons located there are activated. Dysregulation here could result in causalgia (51) with burning pain, trophic changes (glossy skin) and often a local rise in temperature. If left untreated, hyperalgesia occurs, muscles become fibrosed, osteoporosis develops and there may occur accompanying emotional symptoms.

Livingston (51) pointed out that, "In many of the causalgic sites which have long been established, the higher centers become affected and all manner of physiologic and even organic changes may take place in parts of the body far removed from the original focus of irritation." In some clinical syndromes there may be a combination of somatic, visceral, and psychic irritation, each contributing to the central process. Once a vicious cycle is established, the process tends to become self-sustaining.

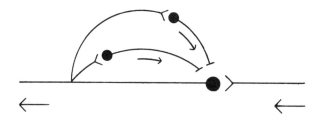

Figure 17. Schematic of reverberating neurone circuits in the central nervous system.

Other post-traumatic pain syndromes as described by Livingston (51) include a peculiar distribution of pain. He speaks of "mirror image" pain in which pain develops in the non-involved side at the precise mirrored location of the contralateral lesion. Such phenomena are explained by the spread of uncontrolled pain by neurons crossing the midline or by spread of excitation by neurohumors to involve other neuron galaxies in the spinal cord within the same segment but on the opposite side. Livingston has also emphasized the importance of recognizing neurotome distribution which can be an important principle in acupuncture treatment. An example is his "multifidus triangle syndrome." Here, the innervation of the multifidus muscle by S1-3 may refer pain to both the lateral thigh and the sciatic distribution in the lower leg.

The term, "pain memory," has been utilized by Melzack and others to describe long-term chronic pain. The intensity of such chronic pain may gradually abate under the application of repeated acupuncture treatments given over a period of days or weeks. This physiologic effect could thus result from a kind of kindling of activity that inhibits the reverberating pain circuits, or it may be that repeated acupuncture treatments stimulate those neurochemical pain control mechanisms that somehow had been lulled into relative inactivity. Acupuncture stimuli then bring new life, as it were, into nature's own mechanism for the release of pain-inhibiting neurohumors.

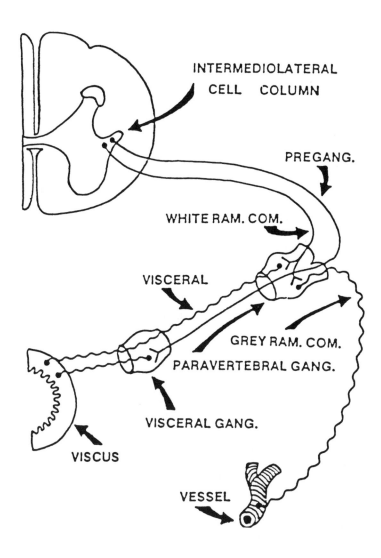

Figure 18. Relationship of the sympathetic nervous system to the intermediolateral cell column of the spinal cord.

BIBLIOGRAPHY

1. Han JS: *The Neurochemical Basis of Pain Relief by Acupuncture. A Collection of Papers* 1973-1987. Beijing, China, Beijing Medical University, 1987.

2. Research Group of Acunpuncture Anesthesia, Peking Medical College: The role of some neurotransmitters of the brain in finger-acupuncture analgesia. **Sci Sin 17**:1123-130, 1974.

3. Myers RD: Transfusion of cerebrospinal fluid and tissue bound chemical factors between the brains of conscious monkeys: a new neurobiological assay. **Physiol Behav 2**:373-377, 1967.

4. Research Group of Acupuncture Anesthesia, Peking Medical College: The effect of PCP and 5-HTP on acupuncture analgesia in the rat. **J New Med Pharmacol 3**:133-138, 1976.

5. Han JS, Chou PH, Lu CC, Lu LH, Yang TS, Jen MF (Research Group of Acupuncture Anesthesia, Peking Medical College): The role of central 5-hydroxytryptamine in acupuncture anaglesia. **Sci Sin 22**:91-104, 1979.

6. Cheng R, Pomeranz B: A combined treatment with D-amino acids and electro-acupuncture produces a greater anesthesia than either treatment alone: naloxone reverses these effects. *Pain* 8:231-236, 1980.

7. Ehrenpreis S: Analgesic properties of enkephalinase inhibitors: animal and human studies. **Prog Clin Res 192**:363-370, 1985.

8. Kaada B, Jorum E, Sagvolden T: Analgesia induced by trigeminal nerve stimulation (electro-acupuncture) abolished by nuclei raphe lesions in rats. **Acupunct Electrother Res 4**:221-234, 1979.

9. Shimizu T, Koja T, et al: Effects of methysergide and naloxone on analgesia produced by peripheral electrical stimulation in mice. **Brain Res 208**:463-467, 1981.

10. Xie GX, Han JS, Hoolt V: Electroacupuncture analgesia blocked by microinjection of anti-beta-endorphin antiserum into periaqueductal grey of the rabbit. **Int J Neurosci 18**:287-291, 1983.

11. Cheng R, Pomeranz B: Monoaminergic mechanisms of electroacupuncture analgesia. **Brain Res 215**:77-92, 1981.

12. Hammond DL: Pharmacology of central pain modulating networks (biogenic amines and non-opioid analgesics). In Fields H, Dubner R, Cervero F(eds): **Advances in Pain Research and Therapy** . New York, Raven Pres, 1985, vol 9, pp 499-511.

13. Chang HT: Integrative action of thalamus in the process of acupuncture for analgesia. **Sci Sin 16**:25-60, 1973.

14. Mayer DJ, Price DD, Raffii A: Antagonism of acupuncture analgesia in man by the narcotic antagonist naloxone. **Brain Res 121**:368-373, 1977.

15. Zhou ZF, Du MY, Han JS: *et al:* Effect of intracerebral microinjection of naloxone on acupuncture and morphine-analgesia in the rabbit. **Sci Sin** 24:1166-1178 1981.

16. Han JS, Xie GX, Zhou ZF, Fokesoon R, Terenuius L: Enkephalin and B-endorphin as mediators of electro-acupuncture analgesia in rabbits. An antiserum microinjection study. **Adv Biochem Psychopahrmacol** 33:369-377, 1982.

17. Han JS, Xie GX; Dynorphin: important mediator for electro-acupuncture analgesia in the spinal cord of the rabbit. **Pain** 18:367-377, 1984.

18. Han JS, Xie GX, Goldstein A: Analgesia induced by intrathecal injection of dynorphin B in the rat. **Life Sci** 34:1573-1579, 1984.

19. Peets J, Pomeranz, B: CXBX mice deficient in opiate receptors show poor electro-aupuncture analgesia. **Nature** 273:675-676, 1978.

20. Sjolund B, Terenius L, Eriksson M: Increased cerebrospinal fluid levels of endorphins after electro-acupucnture. **Acata Physiol Scand** 100:382-384 1977.

21. Masala A, Satta G, Alagna S, *et al:* Suppression of electro-acupuncture (EA)-induced beta-endorphin and ACTH release by hydrocortisone in man. Absence of effects on EA-induced anethesia. **ACTA Endocrinol (Copenh)** 103:469-472, 1983.

22. Han JS, and Sun SL: Differential Release of Enkephalin and Dynorphin by Low and High Frequency Electroacupuncture in the Central Nervous System. **Acupuncture, The Scientific International Journal.** 1;19-27, 1990.

23. Pomeranz B, Cheng R: Suppression of noxious responses in single neurones of cat spinal cord by electro-acupuncture and its reversal by the opiate antagonist naloxone. **Exp Neurol.** 64:327-341, 1979.

24. Cheng R, Pomeranz B: Electro-acupuncture analgesia could be mediated by at least two pain relieving mechanisms: endorphin and non-endorphin systems. **Life Sci** 25:1957-1962, 1980.

25. Sjolund BH, Erikson BE: The influence of naloxone on analgesia produced by peripheral conditioning stimulation. **Brain Res** 173:295-301, 1979.

26. Pomeranz B: Acupuncture neurophysiology. In Adelman G (ed): **Encyclopedia of Neuroscience.** Birkahuser, Boston, 1986.

27. Watkins LR, Mayer DJ: Organization of endogenous opiate and non-opiate pain control systems. **Science** 216:1192-2285.

28. Han JS: Progress in the pharmcological studies of acupuncture analgesia. In Paton SW, Mitchell J, Turner P (eds): **Proceedings IUPHAR Ninth International Congress of Pharmacology.** London, Macmillan, 1984. vol 1, pp. 387-394.

29. Han JS, Ding XZ, Fan SG: Cholecystokinin octapeptide (CCK-8): antagonism to electro-acupuncture analgesia and a possible role in electro-acupuncture tolerance. Pain 27:101-115, 1986.

30. Melzack, R., Wall, P. : Pain Mechanism; A New Theory. Science 1965. 150:971-973.

31. Han, CS, Tang. J., Jen, MF., Zhou, AF., Fan, SC., and Qio XC.: The role of central neurotransmitter in acupuncture analgesia. Private Publication. Research Group of Acupuncture Anesthesia. Peking, People's Republic of China.

32. Han JS, Yu LC, Shi YS: A mesolimbic loop of analgesia. III. A neuronal pathway from nucleus accumbens to periaqueductal grey. Asian Pacific J. Pharmacol 1:17-22, 1986.

33. Bloom R, Guillermin R, et al: Neurons containing B-endorphin in rat brain exist separately from those containing enkephalin: immuno-cytochemical studies. Proc Natl Acad Sci (USA) 765:1591-1595, 1978.

34. Watson SJ, Barchas JD: Anatomy of the endogenous opioid peptides and related substances. In Beers RF (Ed.): Mechanisms of Pain and Analgesic Compounds. New York, Raven Press, 1979, pp. 227-237.

35. Sato T, Usami S, Takeshige C: Role of the arcuate nucleus of the hypothalamus as the descending pain inhibitory system in acupuncture point and non-point produced analgesia (in Japanese, English summary). In Takeshige C (Ed.): Studies on the Mechanism of Acupuncture Analgesia Based on Animal Experiments. Tokyo, Showa University Press, 1986, p. 627.

36. Rossier J, Guillemin R, Bloom FE: Foot shock-induced stress increases B-endorphin levels in the blood but not brain. Nature 270:618-620, 1977.

37. Peng TC and Greenfield W: A Precise Scientific Explanation of Acupuncture Mechanisms: Are We On the Threshold? An Editorial Review. Acupuncture, the International Scientific Journal. 1:28-29, 1990.

38. Melzack R, Melinkoff RF: Analgesia produced by brain stimulation. Evidence of a prolonged onset period. Exp Neruol 43:369-374, 1974.

39. Shyu BC, Andersson SA, Thoren P: Endorphin mediated increase in pain threshold induced by long-lasting exercise in rats. Life Sci 8:833-840 1982.

40. Roos A, Rydenhag C, Andersson SA: Activity in cortical cells after stimulation of tooth pulp afferent in the cat. Extracellular analysis. Pain 16:49-60, 1983.

41. Roos A, Rydenhag, B, Andersson SA: Cortical responses evoked by tooth pulp stimulation in the cat. Pain 3:247-265, 1982.

42. Rydenhag B, Olausson B, Andersson, SA: Projection of tooth pulp afferents to the thalamus of the cat. I. Focal potentials and thalamocortical connections. Exp Brain Res 64:37-48, 1986.

43. Rydenhag B, Olausson B, Shyu BC, Andersson S: Localized responses in the midsuprasylvian gyrus of the cat following stimulation of the central lateral nucleus in thalamus. Exp Brain Res 623:11-24, 1986.

44. Peking Acupuncture Anesthesia Coordinating Group: Preliminary study of the mechanism of acupuncture anesthesia. Sci Sin 16:447-456, 1973.

45. Lassen NA, Ingvar DH, Skinh JE: Brain function and blood flow. Sci Am 239;62-71, 1978.

46. Hand PF, Juang YH, Liu CN: Use of the ($_{14}$C)- deoxyglucose method in acupuncture analgesia studies (abstract). Acupunct Electrother Res 10 (4):364, 1985.

47. Gaito J: The kindling effect. Physiol Psychol 2:45-50, 1965.

48. Lorente de No R: Analysis of the activity of chains of internucial neurons. J Neurophysiol 1:207-244, 1938.

49. Dusser de Barenne JG, McCulloch WS: Factors for facilitation and extinction in the central nervous system. J Neurophysiol 2:319-355, 1939.

50. Loeser JD, Ward AA, White LE: Chronic deafferentation of human spinal cord neurons Neurosurg 29:48-50, 1968.

51. Livingston WK: Pain Mechanisms. New York Macmillan, 1943, p. 253.

Chapter V

NEEDLING POINTS AND TREATMENT STRATEGIES

By tradition, there are some 360 acupuncture points. Over the centuries, practitioners, for whatever reasons, added other points. The expansion of auriculotherapy, the advent of acupuncture "anesthesia" and the recent rebirth of interest in acupuncture throughout the world have, altogether, resulted in an increase of points used over the body until the number described to date reaches 1,000. Once the approximate location of the point had been decided upon, it was stated that careful palpation could reveal a slight depression in the subcutaneous tissue. Some points were said to be tender to pressure, others were felt as nodules.

Useful acupuncture may be practiced with knowledge of the location of only 50-75 physiologically active points. Most of such useful points coincide with motor points and lie close to nerve trunks or Golgi tendon organs. In principle, points for effective stimulation lie within the domain of the neurotome corresponding to the area of disturbance and as such are capable of evoking changes in visceral as well as somatic tissues. Those points that are tender or nodular-like are often trigger points.

Originally such physiologically active points as described above were discovered serendipitously. They became enshrouded in the meridian theory and were soon lost among dozens of other lesser or inactive points that became incorporated into traditional acupuncture theory over the centuries. It has only been recently that the more active acupuncture points were found to coincide with known motor points or nerve trunk locations.

Our own work (1), has demonstrated that many of these points have a strong electrical potential, positive or negative and up to 42 millivolts. Such electrical identity has led to the development of electrical point locators that operate on the basis of lowered skin resistance. These instruments utilize a roving electrode with a ground electrode and permit the passage of a small electrical current to measure local changes in skin resistance. Either a movement of the indicator on a meter or a change in sound from a small speaker demonstrates the different resistance of an "active" point. Repeated measurement, changes in pressure on the electrodes, sweating, etc., can cause false measurement, and hence, this system of point location is fraught with considerable error.

54

The basic principle of point selection for needle placement may be most simply expressed as locating an area of the body where stimulation will produce a beneficial change in the central nervous system through a modulation of ongoing activity. Such points usually lie within or near the neural segment that supplies innervation to the afflicted area. Needle placement should, therefore, be in a motor point, as determined from anatomical charts, adjacent to a major afferent nerve, within a neural plexus, at a trigger point or at a neurotome reference point (Fig. 19 a,b). In this way the stimulation permits access to that part of the neuraxis where the noxious disturbance has its origin. Such areas will ordinarily lie within the neurotome (dermatome or myotome) of the troubled area (Fig. 20 a,b).

The hypothesized events that occur following stimulation of such points begin first at the point of entry of the stimulus into the central nervous system. This is, at the spinal cord level, presumably in the substantia gelatinosa where the entering impulses from afferent nerve stimulation of A-delta fibers block the more slowly traveling impulses of nociceptive fibers. Secondly, following such events, impulses ascend to similar gating mechanisms at higher levels in the central nervous system and produce even longer lasting influences upon the neurochemistry of the brain through increasing the production and liberation of pain relieving neuro-transmitting substances including the endorphins. With repeated stimulation there appears to be an interruption and ultimately dissolution of reverberating circuits whose self-repetitive nature is undoubtedly the basis for a continuation of the original pathological pain stimulus. Thus it is our belief from our own observations and the experiences of Mann (2), Gunn (3), and others that in the main, points for treatment may be usefully selected on the basis of such neuro-anatomical and neuro-physiological principles. We will explore the selection of such areas for stimulation in greater detail. We will also present some of the formulae for multiple needle placement that have been handed down through the centuries as points that have been found useful for specific afflictions, emphasizing wherever possible those points which, although originally selected empirically, seem to have some rationale in modern scientific terms. In the main we will stress that the selection of acupuncture points for the treatment of any condition should be based upon producing a stimulus in those areas of the central nervous system which refer to the region of pain or disturbance. Such selection will, therefore, rely primarily upon a knowledge of neurotome distribution rather than any dependence upon traditional acupuncture theory for the location of meridian points.

In addition to the selection of points on a regional basis, depending upon the area of pain or dysfunction, there seems to be a general effect operating regardless of where the needle is placed. Thus, many patients report an overall feeling of relaxation or improvement which can be explained in terms of the humoral theory of acupuncture mechanism (4,5,6).

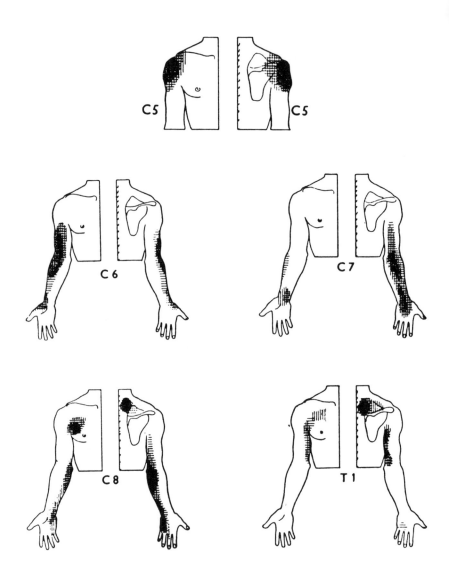

Figure 19a - Distribution of pain on the extremities arising from stimulation of interspinous ligaments C_5, C_6, C_7, C_8, T_1, and L_3, L_4, L_5, S_1 and S_2. From Kellgren, J.K.: On the distribution of pain arising from deep somatic structures with charts of segmental pain areas. *Clinical Science*, 1939-42, 4:35-36.

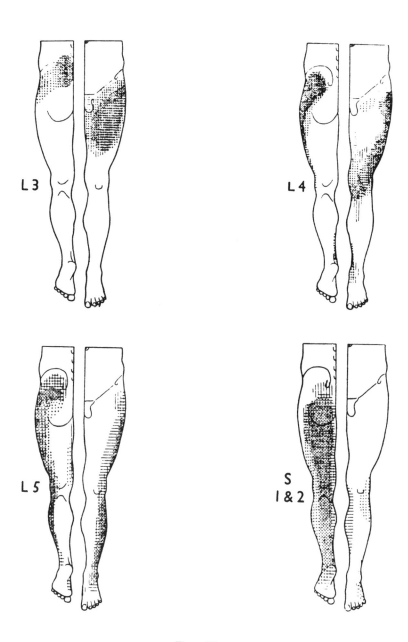

Figure 19b

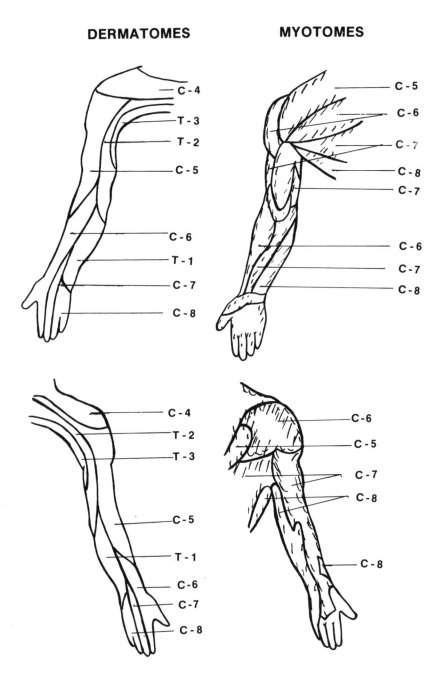

Figure 20a - Comparison of myotome and dermatome distribution from corresponding neurotome segments.

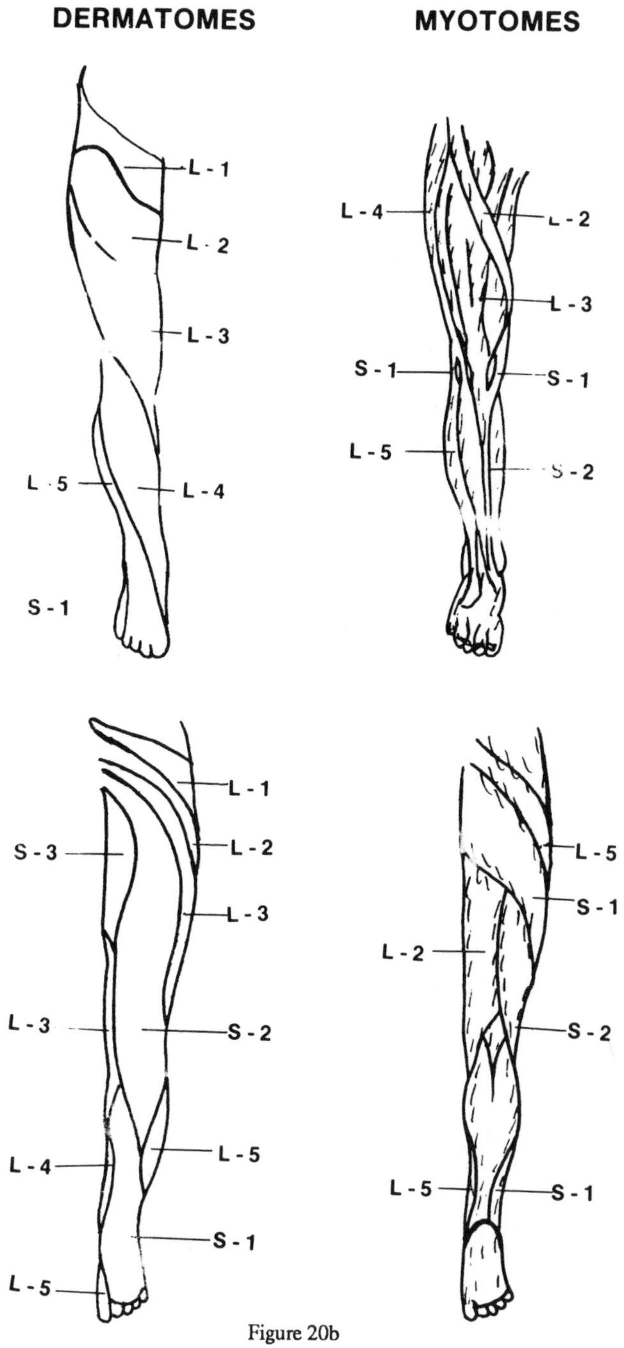

DERMATOMES   **MYOTOMES**

Figure 20b

A. Selection of Motor Points for Stimulation

Recent studies that have compared acupuncture points with motor points (the neurovascular hilus points of electromyography) have found precise concordance in at least 35 points (7, 8). Many other acupuncture points are located close enough to motor points so that electrical stimulation can activate the motor point even when such a point is not in an exactly concordant location. Gunn (3), described some useful acupuncture points located at a focal meeting of superficial nerves in the anterior saggital plane. Other useful points lie over nerve trunks or nerve plexuses. The accompanying Atlas (appendix a-x) refers to points that we have found useful in our clinical practice. The majority of these are motor points, or lie close to the areas where motor points are likely to be found. Thus, in the Atlas figures we have shown the more traditional acupuncture point and, in an adjacent drawing a motor point located nearby. From discussions with traditional Chinese acupuncturists, I have learned that their location of acupuncture points is not an exact science and that even the experts may differ in locating points by several millimeters or perhaps a centimeter or more. We use these listed points for with electrical stimulation, if the needle is located with only approximate accuracy, it simply requires a boost in current to produce an appreciation of the stimulus sensation. A rhythmic pulsation of the needle indicates that efferent motor (muscle) stimulation has been achieved as well as afferent sensory involvement.

We have preserved the original two letter/numerical abbreviation of the meridian designation for those points that are either identical with or lie near motor points. It seemed wise to stay with this traditional designation of acupuncture points as we did not see any gain in confusing an already cluttered literature with yet another system of point nomenclature. Table II lists the abbreviations we have selected to describe the points we use.

B. Selection of Points According to Neurotome Distribution

Previous sections have discussed the Gate theory of Melzak and Wall. The pain mechanisms to be controlled by treatment conceptualized from such a point of view would seem amenable to therapeutic manipulation either within the troubled neurotome or its corresponding myotome, dermatome, sclerotome or sympathetic ramus. It is only necessary to appraise the extent of the pain and locate the appropriate spinal segment involved.

Effective points for the treatment of many conditions, therefore, will be found on the dorsal surface of the body, on either side of the vertebral column, approximately 1-1/2 inches lateral to the midline and at the level of each intervertebral foramen at the point where the spinal nerve exists between the vertebrae (Fig. 21). These correspond approximately to those meridian points called "bladder points" (BL) in traditional Chinese acupuncture (Fig. 22). It is probable that the greatest effect of the simulation here is through muscle afferents of the posterior rami of the spinal nerves. According to the position and depth of placement, needles here will pierce the long muscles of the back (longissimus dorsi and spinalis dorsi) and may reach motor points of the semi-spinalis and multifidus muscles (Fig. 23 a, b, c). Depending upon the strength of electrical stimulus the main entering nerve trunks (posterior and anterior rami), may be stimulated directly. The thickness of the muscle mass here makes it exceedingly unlikely (save with extremely deep penetration) that the peritoneal or thoracic cavities would be inadvertently penetrated.

TABLE II
DESIGNATIONS OF ACUPUNCTURE POINTS USED IN THIS BOOK

Chinese Meridian Abbreviation	Name of Chinese Meridian
LU	Lung
LI	Large intestine
ST	Stomach
SP	Spleen
HE	Heart
SI	Small Intestine
BL	Bladder
KI	Kidney
PC	Pericardium
TH	Triple heater
GB	Gall bladder
LV	Liver
GV	Governing vessel
CV	Conception vessel
EM	"Extra meridian"

Figure 24 illustrates that the palpated vertebral spine does not in all cases correspond to the vertebral body or the spinal nerve root of the same number. It will be recalled that as one descends the spinal cord, the nerve roots angle sharply and must travel longer distances from the shortened cord to the point of their exit from the intervertebral foramina.

Upon entering the spinal cord, afferent impulses from peripheral nerves may synapse directly for reflex arc function or may ascend or descend a few segments. Thus it can often be useful to place needles above or below the neural level of the lesion either to augment the primary stimulus or, when necessary, to avoid a skin area that may be infected, scarred or otherwise inaccessible to use.

Stimulation of the points on the side opposite to the lesion can be effective due to the fact that some fibers cross the spinal cord at or close to the level of the lesion. The ancient acupuncturists took notice of such effects. Thus, there is a saying in the Chinese literature on acupuncture that states: "shoot a bow to the right and to the left to send two arrows at the same time," Such stimulation can be blocked by lesions of the cord, for in hemiplegic patients stimulation of LI-

4 and ST-36 on the side of the lesion failed to produce the rise in pain threshold seen following stimulation of corresponding points on the normal side (9). A similar mechanism in patients with paraplegia blocked the analgesic effect of stimulation at ST-36 on the legs while this lesion did not interfere with the effect of stimulating LI-4 on the hands.

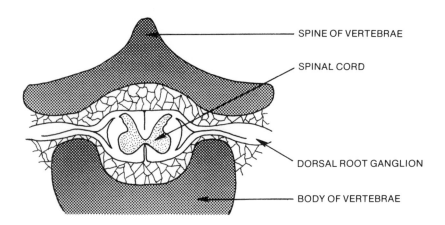

SPINE OF VERTEBRAE

SPINAL CORD

DORSAL ROOT GANGLION

BODY OF VERTEBRAE

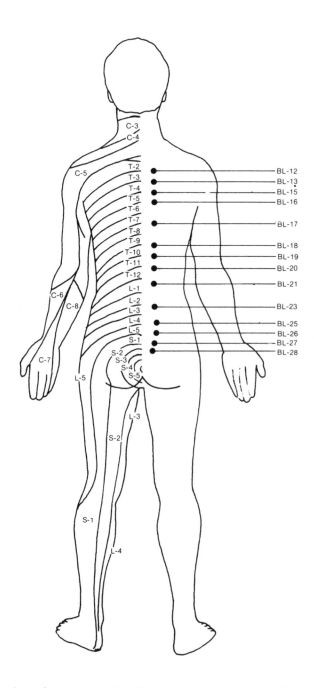

Figure 22 - Correspondence of acupuncture meridian "bladder" points to spinal neurotome distribution.

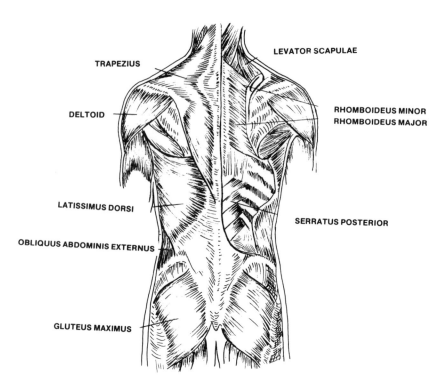

TRAPEZIUS

LEVATOR SCAPULAE

DELTOID

RHOMBOIDEUS MINOR
RHOMBOIDEUS MAJOR

LATISSIMUS DORSI

OBLIQUUS ABDOMINIS EXTERNUS

SERRATUS POSTERIOR

GLUTEUS MAXIMUS

SUPERFICIAL AND INTERMEDIATE MUSCLES OF THE BACK

Figure 23a

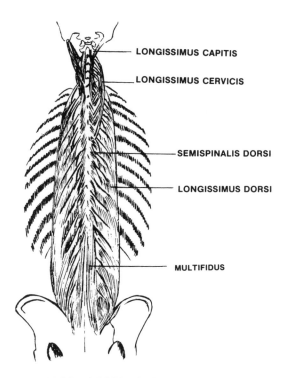

LONGISSIMUS CAPITIS

LONGISSIMUS CERVICIS

SEMISPINALIS DORSI

LONGISSIMUS DORSI

MULTIFIDUS

DEEP MUSCLES OF THE BACK

Figure 23b

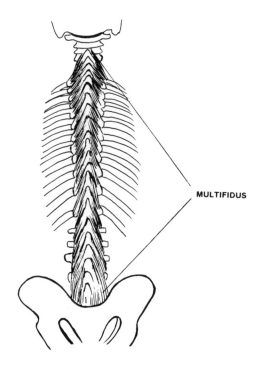

MULTIFIDUS

DEEP MUSCLES OF THE BACK

Figure 23c

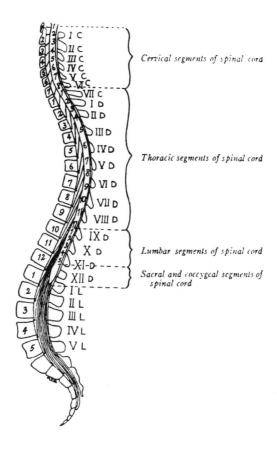

Figure 24 - Level of various segments of the spinal cord with reference to the vertebrae. From Ranson, S.W.: *The Anatomy of the Nervous System*. Sixth Edition, Revised 1939. Saunders Publishing Company.

The importance of segmental neurotome relations has been well illustrated by Chang of Shanghai (10). He demonstrated that stimulation of an acupuncture point which lies at the midpoint of the sterno-cleido-mastoid muscle (also its motor point), produces analgesia sufficient for thyroidectomy. This occurs because this cervical nerve (C3) is from the same spinal root that serves the capsule of the thyroid gland. The same principle can apply to treatment of the face where areas supplied by sensory innervation distributed over the three branches of the trigeminal nerve, ophthalmic, maxillary and mandibular (Fig. 25a), may be affected by stimulation of cervical nerve roots. This is possible because the spinal tract of the trigeminal nucleus reaches downwards to meet ascending impulses from the cervical area (25b).

Figure 26 is a diagram illustrating how neurotomes may overlap. Figure 27 a,b, shows diagrams of the neurotome distribution on the surface of the body together with comparable illustrations of dermatome distribution. This makes it clear why an area painful to deep pressure may relate to the spinal segment innervating the underlying muscle (myotome), rather than the spinal segment overlying the afflicted spot (dermatome). It may be appropriate to place a needle for stimulation in the tender area or motor point of the affected muscle and, as well, in the paravertebral point of the corresponding neurotome. Such needles should be placed deeply within the muscle tissue. It has long been noted in the acupuncture literature that the most effective treatment occurs when the needle is placed to such depth that needle sensation (a dull ache, throbbing or drawing sensation) is experienced. This, commonly known as the "Teh Ch'i" phenomenon, occurs as a result of stimulation of muscle mechanoreceptors (11).

At times, it may be appropriate to place needles more superficially to stimulate tender points within the skin or subcutaneous tissue (dermatomes). Electrical stimulation of such dermatome points can also produce a counter-irritant effect as seen with light stimulation using the flat, superficially applied conductive polymer electrodes of TENS (transcutaneous nerve stimulation). For some patients and for some conditions, deeper motor point stimulation by needles may be preferable to stimulation by surface electrodes.

C. Cutaneo-Visceral and Viscero-Cutaneous Reflex Points

Paralleling the paradigm for selection of points for stimulation within neural segments for referred pain from musculo-fascial structures is that for locating points for the treatment of visceral dysfunction. Such points of reference have long been known in medicine. Henry Head, in 1893 (12), noted the cutaneously referred pain of visceral disease. He demonstrated that counter irritation over the skin and subcutaneous areas of maximal tenderness could alleviate visceral disturbances. He noted that there was often a bilateral distribution of the pain, especially with chronic visceral disturbances. MacKenzie (13), and Kellgran (14), have shown that pain arising from viscera will call into play

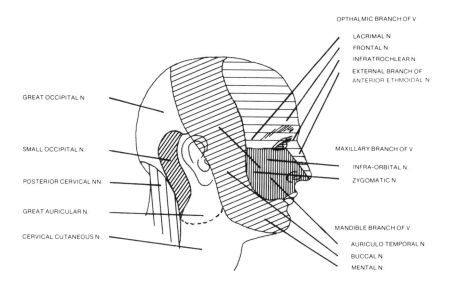

Figure 25a - Sensory zones of the head and neck.

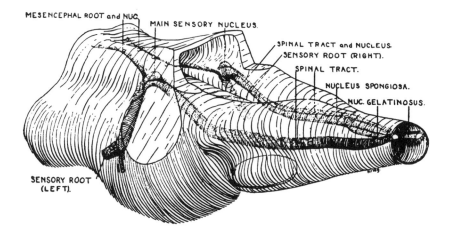

Figure 25b - Location of trigeminal, spinal 5th nucelus in brain stem and upper cervical cord. From Krieg, Wendell, J.S.: *Functional Neuroanatomy.* McGraw Hill, New York, Second Edition, 1953.

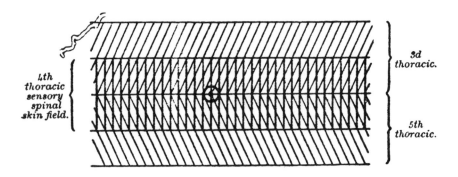

Figure 26 - Schematic illustrating the overlap of dermatomes. From Ranson, S.W.: *The Anatomy of the Nervous System*. Sixth Edition. Revised, 1939. Saunders Publishing Company.

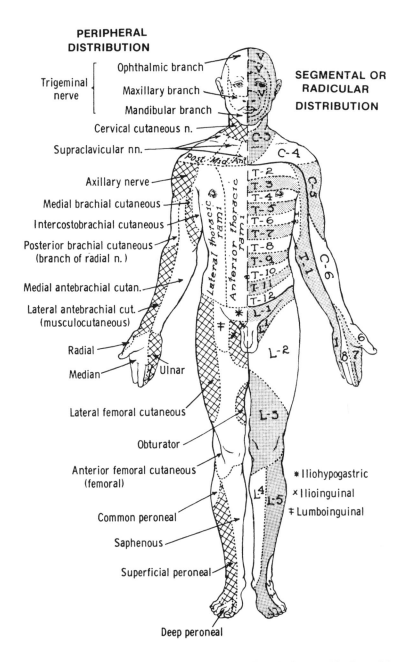

Figure 27a - Neurotome distribution on the human body. From McDonald, J.J., Green, J.R., and Lange, J.: *Correlative Neuroanatomy*. Third Edition, 1938. University Medical Publishers, Palo Alto, Ca.

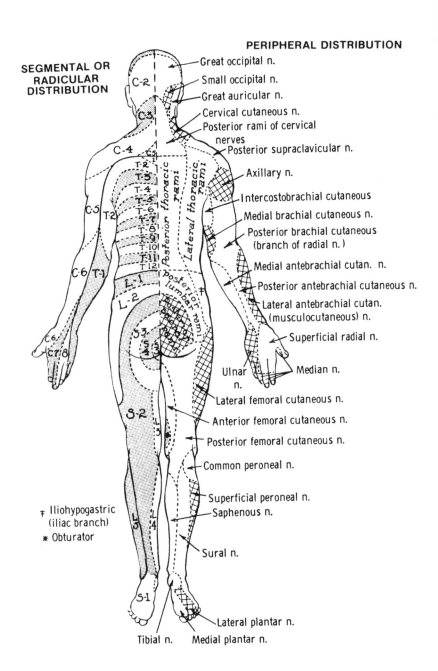

SEGMENTAL OR RADICULAR DISTRIBUTION

PERIPHERAL DISTRIBUTION

Great occipital n.

Small occipital n.

Great auricular n.

Cervical cutaneous n.

Posterior rami of cervical nerves

Posterior supraclavicular n.

Axillary n.

Intercostobrachial cutaneous

Medial brachial cutaneous n.

Posterior brachial cutaneous (branch of radial n.)

Medial antebrachial cutan. n.

Posterior antebrachial cutaneous n.

Lateral antebrachial cutan. (musculocutaneous) n.

Superficial radial n.

Ulnar n.

Median n.

Lateral femoral cutaneous n.

Anterior femoral cutaneous n.

Posterior femoral cutaneous n.

Common peroneal n.

Superficial peroneal n.

Saphenous n.

Sural n.

Lateral plantar n.

Tibial n.   Medial plantar n.

≠ Iliohypogastric (iliac branch)
∗ Obturator

Figure 27b

the cerebrospinal system of sensory nerves with the pain being referred reflexly to the area supplied by the corresponding neurotome. Mann (2), early used the concept of viscero-cutaneous and cutaneo-visceral points to describe the action of some acupuncture points on organs. Weiss and Davis in 1928 (15), noted that referred pain from internally located viscera could be abolished by procaine infiltration of tender areas in the somatic zones of reference, zones that followed patterns often highly consistent from one person to another. Thus, for practical purposes, the segmental distribution of nerves may be of use in selecting effective points for stimulation for the relief of visceral dysfunction.

As disease modifies the function of one organ it may well also affect other organs. This is not only because their functions may interrelate, but also because of the spread of neural irritation to adjacent segments up and down the spinal cord. Thus, for example, pain, muscular contractions and vomiting can occur from disturbance of the viscera at any of several locations in the body. The segment of spinal cord stimulated by the afferent autonomic fibers from the disturbed viscus can become irritable and produce pain, as well as hyperalgesia of both the skin and the muscles in the external body wall. The area may be remote from the disturbed viscus, lie over it or extend widely around it, but in all cases reference to neurotome locations can serve to identify the point for stimulation.

In the living organism there is a succession of stimuli constantly passing from the viscera via afferent nerves to the spinal cord and producing a reflex regulation to maintain homeostasis in muscles, blood vessels, etc. These processes are continually conducted and in such a way that they give rise to no appreciable sensation. If, however, some morbid process occurs in any viscus an imbalance may occur in the homeostatic mechanism. This can affect neighboring nerve cells and can induce a reaction of increased muscle tension in the corresponding myotome or sensory change in the corresponding dermatome. To restore homeostasis it is suggested that the locus of stimulation be in the dermatome or myotome that corresponds to the nerve supplying the afflicted organ.

Figure 28 shows the correspondence between certain para-vertebrally located acupuncture points and the neurotome segments that innervate body organs. These points (BL points), are ideally situated for stimulation of the dorsal roots carrying afferent impulses from these organs. Figure 29 illustrates the mechanism of referred pain by which a stimulus from a dysfunctioning organ (splanchnotome) enters the spinal cord and appears as an area of pain on the body wall (dermatome), corresponding to the viscera served by this same spinal cord segment (neurotome).

On the face, head and neck areas the same principles may be followed. The Chinese have long used the daily massage of points around the orbit for the promotion of good vision and the treatment of occular problems. The facial point, Ying Hsiang (LI-20), has a clinically demonstrated reflex effect upon the mucous linings of the nasal cavity and has, thus, been useful for the relief of sinus congestion. Its translation, "welcome fragrance," speaks directly of its efficacy. Several points around the external ear are felt to have a reflex action, probably vascular, that may produce some relief from VIIIth nerve afflictions.

Autonomic effects may be achieved by stimulation not only of the corresponding posterior rami but also by reflex action of more distant peripheral points (16). It has been shown by Matsumoto (17), that stimulation of ST-36 can induce peristalsis in post-surgical atony of the gut, both in rabbits and in man. The same point can quiet the increased peristalsis of a colon after the administration of CCK-8. Omura (18), has demonstrated that the stimulation of many acupuncture points can produce effects upon microcirculation. There is initially vasoconstriction followed by a more prolonged vasodilitation. It thus appears evident that referred pain and acupuncture share the same pathways within a single neurotome with the skin (dermatome) at one end and the internal organ (splanchnotome) at the other. Thus when disturbance occurs in an organ, pain can be referred to a corresponding skin area. Acupuncture at this point of maximal tenderness can induce a cutaneovisceral reflex attenutating the referred pain and the visceral disturbance (19).

Ear acupuncture illustrates well the use of cutaneous points to affect visceral function. The ear is innervated by branches derived from the trigeminal nerve, facial, glossopharyngeal, vagus, major auricular nerve and the minor occipital nerve. Of these, the vagus is the most important (Figure 30). Points of low resistance were found in the rabbits ear in the area innervated by auricular branches of the vagus nerve (20). The major basis for the effectiveness of ear acupuncture appears to be the fact that the concha of the ear is the only place on the surface of the body where one can easily stimulate fibers of the vagus nerve (Nerve of Arnold). This nerve reaches many of the major viscera of the body and therefore represents a parasympathetic, homeostatic regulatory mechanism.

D. Trigger Points and Reference Areas of Pain

At times it may be appropriate to select points for acupuncture stimulation according to the localization of trigger point reflex pain areas in the manner of techniques elucidated by Travell (21, 22, 23). She described small hypersensitive loci in the myofascial structures that when stimulated, touched or probed, give rise to a larger area of pain in an adjacent or distant reference area. She noted that such trigger points were more or less constant in their location from one person to another. It will be seen in the accompanying illustrations adapted from her work (Figure 30 a-d). That many of the designated trigger spots were identical or similar in location to some acupuncture points. This concordance of acupuncture points and trigger points has been reported to be as high as 71% (24). Other points could well be the extra meridian sensitive "ouch" spots not infrequently used by acupuncturists in the treatment of pain.

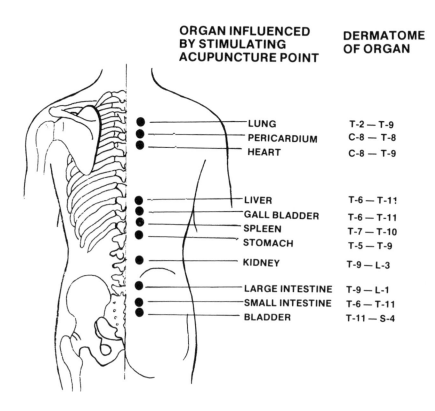

ORGAN INFLUENCED
BY STIMULATING
ACUPUNCTURE POINT

DERMATOME
OF ORGAN

Organ	Dermatome
LUNG	T-2 — T-9
PERICARDIUM	C-8 — T-8
HEART	C-8 — T-9
LIVER	T-6 — T-11
GALL BLADDER	T-6 — T-11
SPLEEN	T-7 — T-10
STOMACH	T-5 — T-9
KIDNEY	T-9 — L-3
LARGE INTESTINE	T-9 — L-1
SMALL INTESTINE	T-6 — T-11
BLADDER	T-11 — S-4

Figure 28 - Correspondence between some para-vertebral acupuncture points and neurotome segments that innervate body organs.

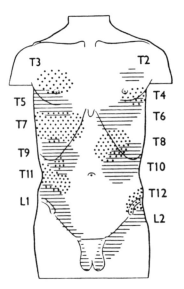 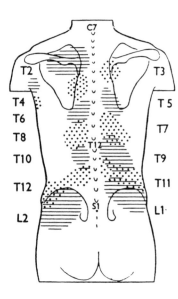

Figure 29 - Distribution of pain on the body wall arising from stimulation of interspinous ligaments. A presumed mechanism for referral of pain from organ dysfunction within the same neurotome. From Kellgren, J.K.: On the distribution of pain arising from deep somatic structures with charts of segmental pain areas. *Clinical Science*, 1939-42, 4:35-36.

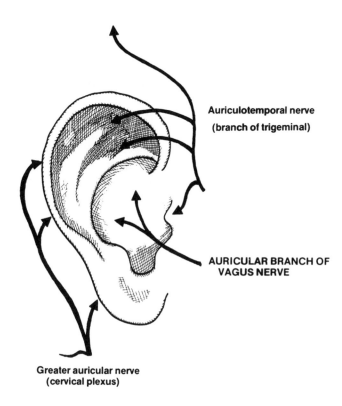

Figure 30 - Innervation of the ear.

Travell has postulated that some initial insult sets in motion a chain of events which is thus perpetuated by a continuing cycle of nerve impulses that have no further dependence upon afferent stimulation, but rather are sustained by facilitation of the noxious stimuli in closed, self re-exciting chains of internuncial neurons in the central nervous system. The initial stimulus can be a direct trauma to the muscle, chronic muscular strain, chilling of fatigued muscles, acute myositis, arthritis, nerve root injury or visceral ischemia. Peripheral factors include fatigue, chronic infection and psychogenic stress. Electro-acupuncture can act presumably by breaking up such reverberating neuronal circuits.

Protracted myofascial pain following pressure upon trigger points is thought to depend on a reflex pain cycle mediated by the trigger area. Travell reported both temporary and permanent relief from chronic myofascial pain by dry needling of these trigger areas. It is of interest that in some of the trigger/reflex areas she observed the symptom pattern could be of a complex nature rather than simple pain. Thus, a trigger spot in the sterno-cleido-mastoid muscle, for example, was described as producing dizziness, imbalance and headaches, with at times nausea, vomiting and tinnitus. She also demonstrated the relief of headaches, breast pain, cardiac pain and other symptoms by needle stimulation of appropriate cutaneous reference zones for such visceral disturbance.

E. SUMMARY-PROCEDURE From the above discussion of motor points, viscero-cutaneous reflexes and trigger points, it can be seen that there are several choices of point selection for electro-acupuncture stimulation. Any of these methods of point selection may be utilized for sequential treatment sessions or selection of several points from each method might be used during a single treatment session. The complex interacting pathways of the central nervous system permit a single point of stimulation to be active in several ways and, as well, for the stimulation of several selected points to effect relief in a single area or an organ system.

Our procedure is to initially search for trigger points. When such a point or points are found, an acupuncture needle is inserted directly and deeply into the muscle tissue in the center of the point. If finger pressure on the point has produced referred pain to another area that area is also so treated. If conductive polymer disc electrodes are used they are placed directly over the point area to be used. In the descriptions here given for needle placement the substitution of disc electrodes will likewise follow the same procedures as given.

Should trigger points not be present, needles are inserted into motor points of the afflicted area as near as possible to the point of pain. With electrical stimulation two needles are required for each stimulating circuit. We usually place an even number of needles, 2, 4, or 6, around the area of pain. The number of needles used depends upon the number of paired lead outlets in the stimulating

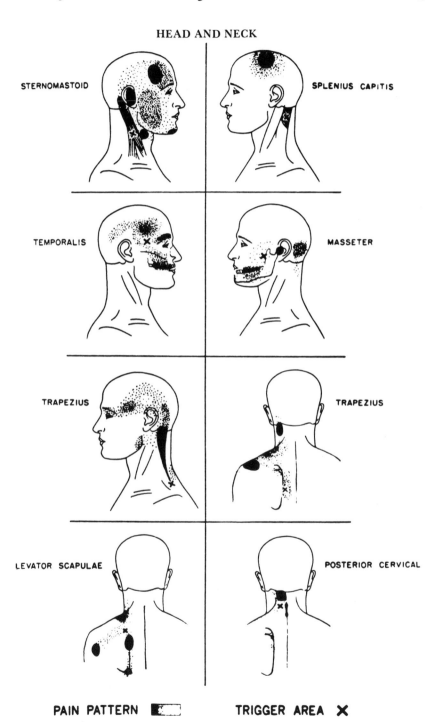

Figure 31a

LOWER EXTREMITY

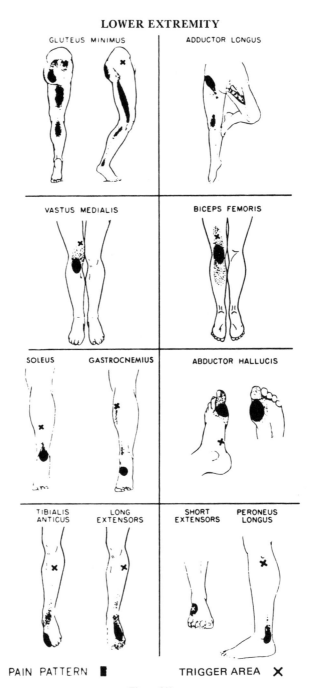

Figure 31b

SHOULDER AND ARM

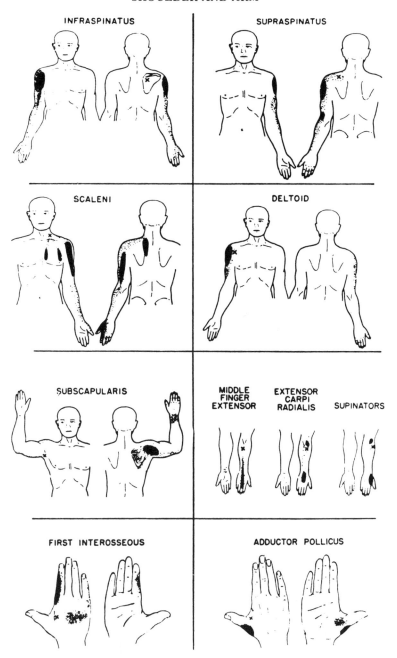

Figure 31c

CHEST AND BACK

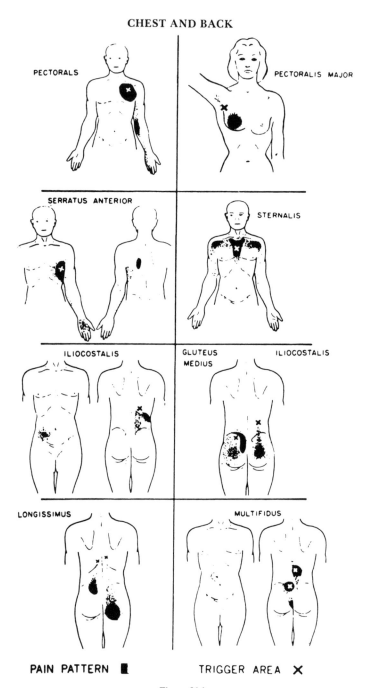

PAIN PATTERN ▮   TRIGGER AREA ✕

Figure 31d

apparatus. It is not necessary that the needles be connected in any particular fashion. For any pair of leads the needles may be far apart in different parts of the body or even on different limbs.

If the affected area does not require or permit the insertion of all needles, some of the needles may be placed in those points located approximately one and one half inches lateral to the spine. The point then selected is close to the exit of the nerve root of the neurotome corresponding to the affected area. If one cannot find a trigger spot or has found the use of trigger spots and/or motor points to be relatively ineffective, it is possible to use only the para-spinal or neurotome (BL) points. Thus, depending upon the progress of the patient, one may from treatment-to-treatment, vary the selection of the points to be used.

In the treatment of conditions other than pain one can use primarily stimulation of the neurotome corresponding to the organ system involved -- again para-spinal points. For psychosomatic conditions and anxiety two needles are used, one in the concha of each ear.

All electrical stimuli are at low frequencies, 2-4 Hertz, alternated with high frequency 80-100 Hertz (dense/disperse current) and with initial adjustment to a level where the patient can just feel the stimulus comfortably or, if in or near a motor point, to an intensity that will cause the needle to vibrate. We do not later increase the current even though the patient may adapt to the stimulus given and report that the current pulses are no longer perceptible. Thus, throughout the treatment, the volume control is not changed. The duration of the stimulation is 30 minutes.

F. SELECTION OF ACUPUNCTURE POINTS BY FORMULA. Contemporary teaching of acupuncture today is usually based on the concept of treatment according to set formulae. There are certain sets of points recommended for use with each specific illness or symptom. A major difficulty with this approach lies in the fact that such formulae have been only empirically determined and their validity as yet untested by scientific means. As one pursues the published literature on acupuncture it becomes quickly evident that there is little agreement on the formulae to be used for most major illnesses. To date, there has been no acceptable research comparing these formulations either as to their validity or reliability.

The reasons for the widespread use of "acupuncture by formulae" are several: **First,** traditional acupuncture point selection is based upon complicated metaphysical theories for balancing an hypothesized disruption of Yin/Yang energy as detected by pulse diagnosis. Although such a fanciful ritual may have been acceptable in pre-scientific times, with increasing knowledge of anatomy and physiology point selection in this manner is scientifically untenable. Those who remain loyal to such traditional metaphysical beliefs use the excuse that "only a few master acupuncturists are capable of using pulse diagnosis" and, hence, acupuncturists of lesser skill must rely upon formulae. **Second,** according to the teachings of the *Nei Ching* (25), acupuncture performed in accordance with the traditional theoretical concepts was of value primarily for the prevention of illness and should therefore be used only before any serious symptoms of disease become manifest. When signs of major illness were obvious, it was traditionally taught that the energy within the meridians at that time exhibited such a state of fluctuating imbalance that accurate pulse diagnosis was impossible and treatment must begin with needle placement designated by formulae. **Third,** with the recent blending of Western medicine and traditional techniques of acupuncture, the diagnosis of disease became increasingly a matter for laboratory methods and Western physical diagnostic techniques. Illnesses are now given diagnostic labels acceptable to international medical terminology. Thus, "energy balancing" receives much less attention and needle placement on meridian points has been increasingly matched to formulae developed from experience and designated as specifically effective for each type of illness as ascertained by Western diagnosis.

The problem then is that of selecting "which formula for which disease?" It becomes evident from even a preliminary scan of the books on acupuncture that the many "experts" have different preferred sets of points for the same illness. In a study of point formulae recommended for headache, Ulett and Johnson reviewed 33 articles from a Medlars search of recent literature (26). They found that there was a great variety of recommendations and, that although most recommendations contained the two points, LI-4 and GB-20, the other points recommended varied greatly from author to author.

Acupuncture was long an unwritten art, teaching passed from father to son with many secret formulations. Master acupuncturists have also been renowned for their special techniques and "miracle cures." Thus, the use of acupuncture by formulae has a long history. Some of these formulae may have been empirically effective simply because the designated points selected happened to lie over physiologically active areas such as motor points or along major nerve trunks. Despite its many contradictions, the method is universally used and thus perhaps worthy of note at this time of flux from the traditional to a more scientifically based procedure. The use of set formulae may be helpful for the beginning practitioner of acupuncture who, when confronted by the first patients, puzzles over optimal needle placement. With experience there is developed one's own set of preferred formulae. Even these, however, will be varied from patient-to-patient and from treatment-to-treatment to meet the slight but significant differences in site of pain, body asymmetries and the like.

In Figure 32 a-f), we show diagrams of a few formulae selected from leading books on the subject. We have attempted to designate points upon which there

Acupuncture Point Formulae
for the Treatment of
Selected Conditions

WRIST AND HAND PAIN

LI-4
LI-11
HE-7
LU-7

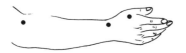

HIP AND LEG PAIN

GB-30
GB-31
GB-34
BL-50
BL-51

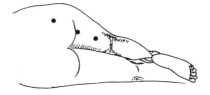

SCIATICA

GB-30
BL-54
BL-25
BL-57
BL-60
BL-23
BL-51

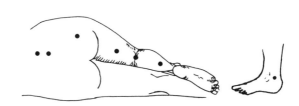

KNEE PAIN

GB-34
SP-10
BL-54
ST-36
ST-32

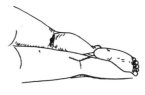

Figure 32a

ANKLE AND FOOT PAIN

BL-60
KI-3
ST-44
LV-3

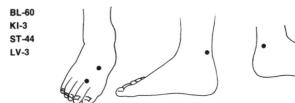

LOW BACK PAIN

INTERCOSTAL NEURALGIA

POST-HERPETIC NEURALGIA

PARAVERTEBRAL POINTS
AT LEVEL OF LESION

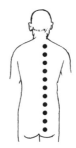

GASTRALGIA

CV-12
BL-21
ST-36
BL-18
LI-4
CV-3
CONCHA OF EAR

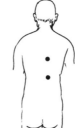

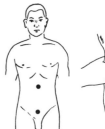

HEMIPLEGIA

LI-16
TH-5
LI-11
LI-4

GB-30
GB-31
GB-34
ST-36
SP-6

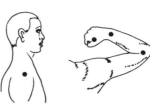

UPPER LIMB

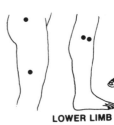

LOWER LIMB

Figure 32b

TEMPORO-MANDIBULAR JOINT PAIN

LI-4
TH-21
SI-19

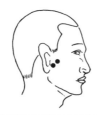

NECK PAIN

GB-20
GB-21
LI-4
TH-14

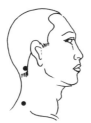

SHOULDER PAIN

LI-14
LI-16
TH-14
GB-21
LI-11
SP-20

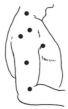

ELBOW PAIN

LI-11
TH-10
LI-4

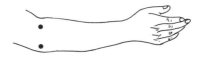

Figure 32c

RHINITIS AND SINUSITIS

GB-20
LI-4
LI-20
BL-2

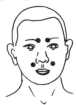 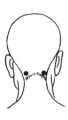

NERVE DEAFNESS
TINNITUS-VERTIGO

ST-7
TH-21
SI-19
TH-17
GB-20

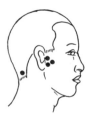

ANXIETY
ASTHMA
HYPERTENSION

CONCHA OF EAR

DEPRESSION

PC-6
ST-36
LI-4
CONCHA OF EAR

 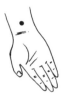 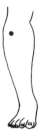 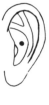

Figure 32d

TOOTHACHE

    LI-4
    ST-7
    ST-6
    ST-4
    ST-5

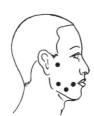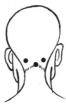

HEADACHE

    GB-20
    LI-4
    EM-1
    GV-20
    GV-15

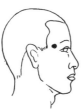

FACIAL PALSY

    BL-2
    ST-4
    LI-4
    ST-7

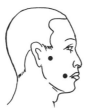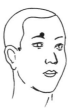

Figure 32e

MENSTRUAL DYSFUNCTION

SP-6
SP-10
CV-3
CV-6

IMPOTENCE

BL-23
BL-50
SP-6
CV-3
ST-36
CONCHA OF EAR

TRIGEMINAL NEURALGIA

TH-21
BL-2   OPHTHALMIC
EM-1

LI-20
GV-26
LI-4   MAXILLARY
ST-1

ST-7
ST-6   MANDIBULAR
ST-4
SI-19

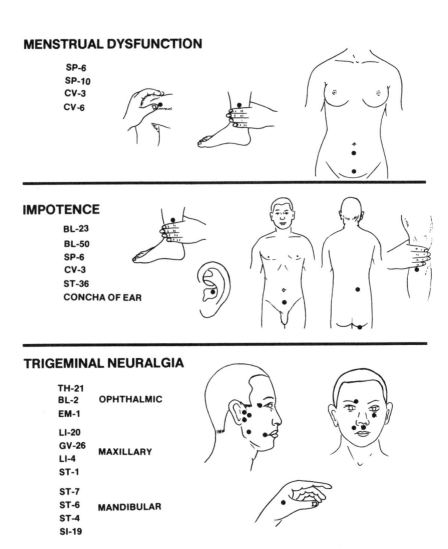

Figure 32f

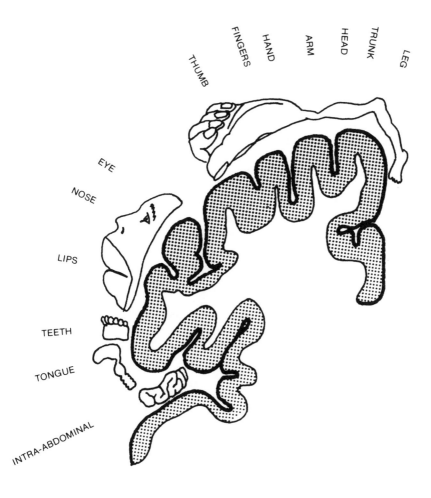

Figure 33

was some agreement among several authors and, as far as possible, points having some physiological rationale for their use.

Although some authorities have listed as many as 20 points for a single condition, we have tried to limit our recommendations to a small number of points for each formula with the suggestion that other regionally appropriate points be added as the variations in location, character and intensity of symptoms are found to vary from patient-to-patient and from one treatment session to another. As experience is gained from the successful treatment of patients, one will feel confident using a smaller rather than a larger number of needles. In view of this, it is interesting to note that a single point, ho ku (LI-4, motor point of the dorsal interosseus and adductor pollicus muscles) is used for afflictions of the upper half of the body. These two muscles are among the most important in the body because the ability to approximate the thumb and index finger have permitted the development of civilization. These muscles are among the most heavily endowed with nerve endings and during early development, when the growing brain exhibits plasticity, the thumb has come to occupy an extremely large area on the surface of the cerebral hemispheres (Fig. 33). Similarly tsu san li (St-36, Motor point of the tibialis anticus), is most commonly used for afflictions of the lower half of the body. Perhaps the above is the basis for a statement in traditional Chinese acupuncture that "the master acupuncturist can cure all illnesses with but a single, well placed needle."

References

1. Brown, MI., Ulett, GA., and Stern, JA: Acupuncture Loci: Techniques for Location. **Amer. J. Chinese, Med**, 2(1) 67-74, 1974.

2. Mann, F.: **Scientific Aspects of Acupuncture.** William Heinemann Medical Books, Ltd. London, 77, 1977.

3. Gunn, CC.: Type IV Acupuncture Points *Am. J. Acupuncture* 5:51-58.

4. Mendelson, G.: Acupuncture Analgesia. II. Review of Current Theories. **Aust., N.Z.J. Med.,** 89:100-105, 1978.

5. Anon: The Relation Between Acupuncture Analgesia and Neurotransmitters in Rabbit Brain. **China Med. J.,** 8:105, 1973

6. Reiderer, P., Tenk, H., Werner, H., Bischko, J., Rett, A., and Krisper, H.: Manipulation of Neurotransmitters by Acupuncture. **J. Neural Transmission,** 37:81, 1975.

7. Liu, YH., Varela, M., Oswald.: The Correspondence Between Some Motor Points and Acupuncture Loci. **Amer. J. Chinese Med.,** 3:347-358, 1975

8. Liao, S.J.: Acupuncture Points. Concordance with Motor Points of Skeletal Muscles. **Arch. Phys. Med. Rehab.,** 56:550, 1975

9. Chang, CY., Chang, CT., *et al.:* Peripheral Efferent Pathways for Acupuncture Analgesia. **Scientia Sineca,** 16:210-217, 1973.

10. Chang, Hsiang-tung: **Peoples Republic of China Acupuncture Anesthesia.** Colored Movies, 1973.

11. Gunn, CC.: Transcutaneous Neural Stimulation, Needle Acupuncture and 'Teh Ch'i' Phenomenon. *Am. J. Acupuncture.* 4:317-322, 1976.

12. Head, H.: On Disturbances of Sensation with Especial Reference to the Pain of Visceral Diseases. **Brain,** 16:1-133, 1893.

13. MacKenzie, J.: **Symptoms and Their Interpretation.** Shaw and Sons, London, p. 304, 1912.

14. Kellgren, JH.: On the Distribution of Pain Arising From Deep Somatic Structures with Charts of Segmental Pain Areas. **Clin. Sci.,** 4:35-46, 1939-42.

15. Weiss, S., and Davis, D.: Significance of Afferent Impulses from Skin in Mechanism of Visceral Pain: Skin Infiltration as Useful Therapeutic Measure. **Amer. J.M. Sci.** 176:51736, 1928.

16. Chang, HT.: Integrative Action of Thalamus in the Process of Acupuncture for Analgesia. **Scientia Sinica,** 16:25-60, 1973.

17. Matsumoto, T.: **Acupuncture for Physicians.** CC Thomas, Springfield, IL. pp. 204, 1974.

18. Omura, Y.: Patho-Physiology of Acupuncture Treatment: Effects of Acupuncture on Cardiovascular and Nervous Systems. **Acupuncture and Electro-Therap. Res. J.** 1:51-140, 1975.

19. Acupuncture Anesthesia Research Group, Morphology Unit, Peking Medical College, Peking Survey of Electric Resistance of Rabbitt's Pinna in Experimental Peritonitis and Peptic Ulcer. **Chinese Med. J., New Series:** 2:423-434, 1976.

20. Liao, SJ.: Recent Advances in Understanding of Acupuncture. **Yale J. Biol. and Med.,** 51:55-65, 1978.

21. Travell, J., and Rinzler, S.H.: Relief of Cardiac Pain by Local Block of Somatic Trigger Areas. **Proc. Soc. Exptl. Biol. Med.,** 63:480-482, 1946.

22. Travell, J: **The Myosfascial Genesis of Pain.** Scientific exhibit shown at Annual Session of American Medical Association, Atlantic City., 1951. Postgrad. Med., 2:425-434, 1952.

23. Travell, JG and Simons, DG.: **Myofascial Pain and Dysfunction.: The Trigger Point Manual.** Vols. 1 1983, Vol. 2, 1991. Williams and Wilkins N.Y.

24. Melzack, R., Stillwell, DM., and Fox, IJ: Trigger Points and Acupuncture Points for Pain: Correlation and Implications. **Pain,** 3:3-23, 1977.

25. Wu Wei-Ping: **Chinese Acupuncture.** Translation by Philip M. Chancellor, Health Science Press, Rustington, Sussex, England, pp. 181, 1959.

26. Ulett G. and Johnson, M.: **Treatment of Headache, Two Kinds of Acupuncture.** In Press.

Chapter VI

TREATMENT TECHNIQUE

Although acupuncture means literally "needle penetration," or "needles through the skin," many physicians today are finding that flexible conducting polymer pad electrodes are more comfortable for the patient and may be equally effective. They are simply coated with electrode jelly and taped to the skin. Another electrode has been suggested in the form of a silver disc with a dull pointed protrusion on side (1). Other physicians feel that needles are essential and certainly many patients come for treatment with the fixed idea that only needles can make them well. Therefore, our discussion here will focus on the use of needles.

NEEDLES With the common fear of spreading AIDS and with knowledge that improperly sterilized needles have indeed been responsible for the spread of hepatitis (2) it is today mandatory that acupuncture be done with disposable needles. These needles come variously packaged. A common type is a pre-sterilized needle contained in its own plastic tube. The needle is slightly longer than the tube in which it is encased (Fig. 33). A slight twist of the protruding top breaks the needle loose from it's seal. The tube is then pressed over the point to be stimulated. A sharp tap of the finger causes the needle to painlessly penetrate the skin. The tube is then removed and the needle twisted and pushed deeper into the muscle tissue.

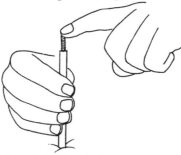

Figure 33. Hollow tube method of inserting fine Japanese acupuncture needles.

There is little or no pain associated with proper needle technique The more rapid the insertion the better. The fingers and skin area to be penetrated should be cleansed with alcohol prior to needle insertion. The depth of insertion must be governed by the size of the muscle mass to be penetrated in order to reach the area of stimulation. It is not possible to give a figure for the safe depth of insertion at each point because there is so much variation from one person to another. A sound knowledge of anatomy is therefore necessary for the proper practice of acupuncture. In this regard a study of cross-sectional anatomy can be helpful (Fig. 34 a, b, c). Whenever possible the tip of the needle should approximate the motor point. When the point is reached the patient may experience a feeling of pressure, heavy soreness or distention. Such sensations are termed "De Qi," or "Teh Ch'i." This awareness of the needle is usually not described as painful. It results from stimulation of the receptors in the muscle, including those nerves involved in proprioception and mechano-reception. This sensation occurs within a few seconds of insertion and may remain localized or can spread along the distribution of the nerve trunk. It is then experienced as a brief "electrical shock."

Most needles are inserted vertically at 90 degrees perpendicular to the skin. In order to bypass certain bones and organs, a 45 degree angle of insertion may sometimes be necessary. For points about the face and head, needles are inserted under, and even more parallel to the skin surface.

COMPLICATIONS. Acupuncture is a very safe method of treatment. Complications and side effects are less than those seen with the administration of pain-killing drugs. If general precautions are taken no complications occur. However, because acupuncture is often done by persons with no medical training, the literature describes a number of instances of untoward happenings.(3)

Dizziness and circulatory shock (fainting) can occur, especially in persons receiving acupuncture for the first time. This may be due to emotional stress, tension, fatigue, hunger, or a labile autonomic nervous system. Be wary of patients who are highly neurotic or who experience profuse sweating and tachycardia and have a weak, thready pulse. Such patients should lie flat on their back and often for their first treatment, no electricity and only a few needles should be used.

Rarely needle grasp may occur, making it difficult to withdraw the needle. This is due to muscle tension or the gamma reflex and can be overcome by relaxing the patient or by the application of a second needle at an angle and adjacent to the impounded needle.

Should a needle bend, simply change the patient's position and withdraw the needle in the direction of the curve. I have never experienced a broken needle. Such complication was occasionally seen when needles were sterilized and reused without discarding those that became defective. With disposable needles this complication should never occur.

Upon removal of the needles, each point should be carefully inspected for bleeding which may appear even after the delay of a minute or two. Surface bleeding can be seen and controlled by pressure. Small ecchymoses may occur

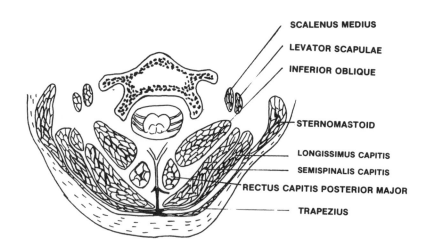

SCALENUS MEDIUS

LEVATOR SCAPULAE

INFERIOR OBLIQUE

STERNOMASTOID

LONGISSIMUS CAPITIS

SEMISPINALIS CAPITIS

RECTUS CAPITIS POSTERIOR MAJOR

TRAPEZIUS

**CROSS-SECTION OF THE NUCHAL REGION AT
THE LEVEL OF THE AXIS**

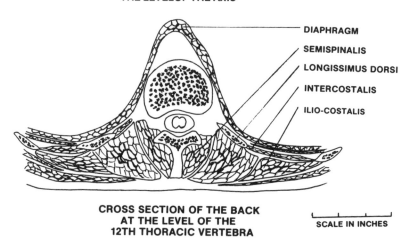

DIAPHRAGM

SEMISPINALIS

LONGISSIMUS DORSI

INTERCOSTALIS

ILIO-COSTALIS

**CROSS SECTION OF THE BACK
AT THE LEVEL OF THE
12TH THORACIC VERTEBRA**

SCALE IN INCHES

Figure 34 a.

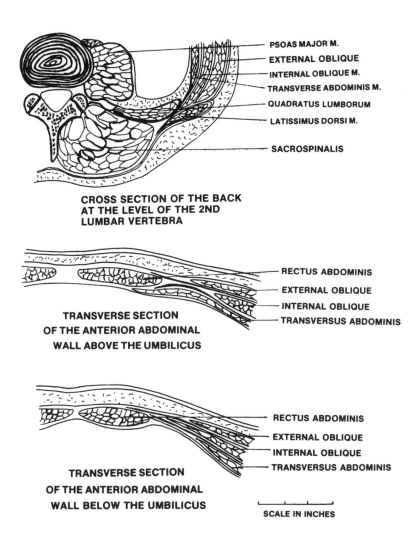

PSOAS MAJOR M.

EXTERNAL OBLIQUE

INTERNAL OBLIQUE M.

TRANSVERSE ABDOMINIS M.

QUADRATUS LUMBORUM

LATISSIMUS DORSI M.

SACROSPINALIS

**CROSS SECTION OF THE BACK
AT THE LEVEL OF THE 2ND
LUMBAR VERTEBRA**

RECTUS ABDOMINIS

EXTERNAL OBLIQUE

INTERNAL OBLIQUE

TRANSVERSUS ABDOMINIS

**TRANSVERSE SECTION
OF THE ANTERIOR ABDOMINAL
WALL ABOVE THE UMBILICUS**

RECTUS ABDOMINIS

EXTERNAL OBLIQUE

INTERNAL OBLIQUE

TRANSVERSUS ABDOMINIS

**TRANSVERSE SECTION
OF THE ANTERIOR ABDOMINAL
WALL BELOW THE UMBILICUS**

SCALE IN INCHES

Figure 34 b.

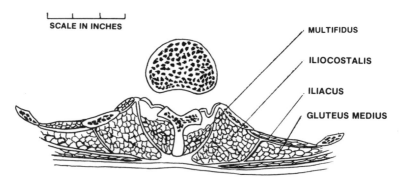

SCALE IN INCHES

MULTIFIDUS

ILIOCOSTALIS

ILIACUS

GLUTEUS MEDIUS

**TRANSVERSE SECTION OF THE BACK AT THE
LEVEL OF THE 5th LUMBAR VERTEBRA**

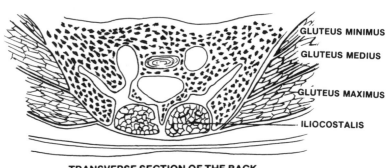

GLUTEUS MINIMUS

GLUTEUS MEDIUS

GLUTEUS MAXIMUS

ILIOCOSTALIS

**TRANSVERSE SECTION OF THE BACK
AT THE LEVEL OF THE
SACRAL PROMONTORY**

Figure 34 c.

some hours later at the point where the needle was inserted. These are of no importance, but the patient should be informed of such possible occurrence. I have treated hemophiliac patients without this complication,

I have never had a single occasion of infection in treating over several thousand patients. With clean technique and the use of disposable needles there should be no occasion for any concern.

In the hands of unskilled practitioners with poor knowledge of anatomy, penetration of organs, especially the intestines, bladder, lungs and peritoneum, has been reported. Atelectasis has been described following treatment of shoulder areas where the acupuncturist has failed to realize that the apex of the left lung in thin females may be within reach of a 2-inch needle. It is therefore important that the selection of needle length should be appropriate to the depth of muscle area to be treated. (Fig. 35). Too shallow penetration is less effective and too deep penetration dangerous. We have found 4 cm. needles to be generally useful with 1.5 cm. preferable about the face and about 60 cm-80 cm. needles useful for the gluteal areas or in heavily muscled or obese patients.

Some pain or discomfort may occur with clumsy, inept techniques or with attempts to insert a bent needle. If the patient moves during or after needle insertion, small muscle tears and pain may result. It is important, therefore that the patient be in a position of comfort for the duration of the treatment. Needling around the face and ear or the tips of the extremities is more painful than elsewhere.

Contraindications to acupuncture include patients who are inebriated and tense or who are perspiring freely. In pregnant women, acupuncture needles should not be inserted in the lumbosacral outflow or on the abdomen below the umbilicus. Electro-acupuncture should not be used near cardiac pacemakers. One should always avoid swollen or infected areas and large blood vessels.

PATIENT SELECTION. I have treated patients of all ages with acupuncture. Although acupuncture is usually given in the physician's office, hospitals are increasingly tolerant of acupuncture procedures. Some insurance companies will reimburse at least in part, for acupuncture, particularly if it is explained in terms of "similar to transcutaneous electrical nerve stimulation."

There is no way to predict which patients will respond to electro-acupuncture stimulation although success on the first treatment may have some positive predictive value. A positive attitude is said to be predictive of successful treatment. but I have found this not to be universally true. I have successfully treated patients who were openly skeptical and who came to the office reluctantly at the urging of a spouse. Less positive results are found with patients who have had previous surgery.

Patients should be psychologically prepared by some discussion of the nature of acupuncture, including the near absence of side effects, no great pain, etc. The use of disposable needles is a great reassurance to many. Patients should be placed in a comfortable position that allows good visual exposure of the part to be treated. They should be cautioned against any gross movements of the body. The bladder should be emptied prior to treatment. They should have no alcohol or drugs active on the nervous system the day prior to treatment.

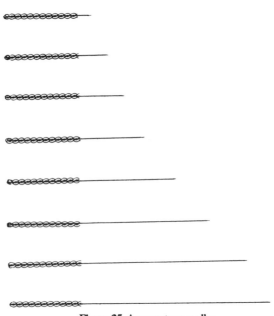

Figure 35. Acupuncture needles.

STIMULATION. Most acupuncture treatment today is accomplished by the use of electrical stimulation (Figure 36). It is certainly easier to apply than manual manipulation. Our studies (4) have shown electrical stimulation to be 100% more effective than simple needling techniques. With electrical stimulation some benefit can be achieved even if the needle is not precisely located because of the spread of the current through the tissues.

The stimulation is brought to the needles by small wire leads from the stimulator, which in turn are attached to the needles by small clips. With conducting polymer electrodes the wires are attached prior to use. The paired wires are usually attached to needles that are nearby each other, although no definite rules have been developed for such selection. The number of points stimulated depends upon the number of lead jacks in the stimulator.

A great deal of investigation remains to be done to ascertain the ideal parameters of stimulation for different types of illness. Currently, it is thought

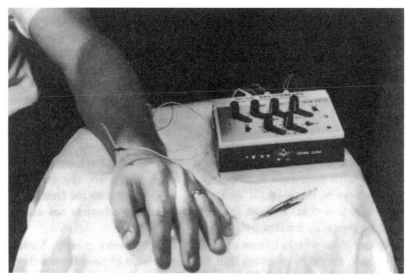

Figure 36. Typical electronic acupuncture stimulator of Chinese manufacture.

that useful stimulation can occur with currents varying from 0.5 to 50 mA. Voltages are from 0.3 to 9 V, usually produced by a 9-V dry cell source. The wave forms vary but customarily are square waves of exponentially rising or falling form and from 0.1 to 0.3 msec. in duration and occurring in trains. Thus, they are pulsating direct current (DC) potentials.

Pulses from 1 to 1000 Hz have been used. Some workers believe that slow pulsations (1-6 Hz) are best for acute pain and fast (80-120 Hz) pulsations are best for chronic pain. This belief is not universally held (5). In all of my treatments I use so called dense-disperse (D-D) stimulation. This has a slow disperse e.g., 2 Hz alternating with a burst of dense (80-100 Hz) waves. In the stimulator we use such alternation occurs at the rate of 2 bursts per second. As it has been shown that too long stimulation at any one frequency can reduce the effectiveness of that frequency, it is felt that alternating the frequencies will maintain each stimulus at maximum efficiency.

Most of the electro-acupuncture equipment on the market produces a square wave output. In this case, the "needle sensation" elicited from the negative electrode is much stronger than that induced from the positive lead.

Polarization may be induced by long term stimulation. To overcome such problems asymmetric, biphasic and modified square wave currents have been used, but these have afforded only a partial solution. We prefer to use the Han-Acutens apparatus (Figure 37) which utilizes identical wave forms with alternating polarity, thus ensuring equally intense stimulation at both electrodes. Most stimulating equipment gives a choice of impulse patterns, with waves being electrode is much stronger than that induced from the positive lead.

Polarization may be induced by long term stimulation. To overcome such problems asymmetric, biphasic and modified square wave currents have been used, but these have afforded only a partial solution. We prefer to use the Han-Acutens apparatus (Figure 37) which utilizes identical wave forms with alternating polarity, thus ensuring equally intense stimulation at both electrodes. Most stimulating equipment gives a choice of impulse patterns, with waves being continuous or coming initially in bursts with the impulse frequency being adjustable. Dense-disperse stimulation may permit either or both frequencies to be adjusted.

Sessions of stimulation may be of any length but it has been shown by Han that the maximum effect is obtained by 30 minutes and after that there is a dropping off of the effect. This probably occurs by reason that CCK-8 is produced and acts as an inhibitory substance. Occasionally, and especially with acute pain, patients will get relief with only one treatment. With chronic pain a number of sessions is usually required. Most reports indicate that improvement will occur with six to eight treatments. Occasionally patients get no therapeutic response until after 10-12 treatments. Initially some patients are treated two or three times a week, later one treatment a week is sufficient. In patients with severe pain, treatment may be given twice a day, although it is important then that several hours elapse between treatments. In other patients e.g., those with chronic arthritis, it has been useful, after an initial course, to continue with maintenance treatments on a once-a-month schedule. I have found that such a schedule may prevent relapse. Other patients obtain complete relief after six or eight treatments and do not require more. Pain relief usually is cumulative with successive treatments, although here too, the course of recovery may be irregular. If there is no sign of relief after 8 to 10 treatments, acupuncture is probably an inappropriate modality for that patient.

The duration of relief from a single treatment varies greatly. Vierck *et al* (6) found in monkeys that suppression of pain from a single treatment could last up to 70 hours, but that the pain threshold showed a major fluctuation during that time. At times, with chronic pain, the greatest relief may appear 1 or 2 days after the treatment. On occasion the pain seems to increase for a few hours following the treatment before a long period of abatement.

The level of stimulation required varies from patient to patient and for the same patient from day to day. The patient should be able to feel the stimulation but it should not be at an uncomfortable level. Often there is muscle fibrillation. The current is adequate when either of the above occurs. As stimulation progresses within a treatment session the patient may state that the stimulus is no longer felt. This is simply the result of body accommodation, the level of stimulation remaining the same. Such accommodation is less likely to occur with

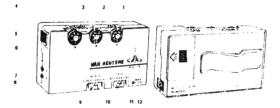

1. Freguency Knob	CONTINUOUS
2. Intensity Knob (CH2)	BURST
3. Intensity Knob (CH1)	D–D(Dense–Disperse)
4. TENS /ACU Switch	10. Power and Output Mode
5. Channel 1 Indicator	OFF (Power off)
6. Channel 1 Output Socket	SYNC (CH1 and CH2 synchronus)
7. Channel 2 Output Socket	ALT (CH1 and CH2 alternate)
8. Channel 2 Indicator	11. BAT LOW (Power Voltage Low Indicator)
9. Waveform Select	12. Adapter Socket

SPECIFICATIONS

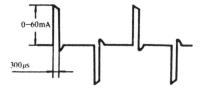

0–60mA

300μs

Amplitude:
Output"ACU": 0–60 mA into 250 ohm load
(for electroacupuncture)
Output"TENS": 0–55 mA into 1 kohm load
(for TENS and SSP)
Pulse width: fixed at 300μs
Frequency range: 2–100 Hz
Impulse pattern:
CONT: Continuous output, frequency 2–100 Hz adjustable
BURST: Intermittent trains of impulses at 2 bursts per second, impulse
frequency 15–100 Hz adjustable

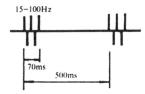

15–100Hz

70ms

500ms

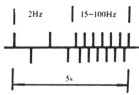

2Hz   15–100Hz

5s

D–D: Dense (15–100 Hz adjustable) and Disperse (2 Hz) impulses appearing
alternatively at 2.5 periods, i.e., 5 s per cycle
Output: Two channel, bipolar output
Input: 9v DC battery (6F22),or External power supply
Dimensions: 122× 88× 26mm
Weight: gm including battery.

Figure 37 HAN-ACUTENS Electro-acupuncture stimulator

the dense-disperse type of stimulating current. In susceptible individuals reddening of the skin can occur even with simple placement of the needle. With careful adjustment of the current there is no discomfort to the patient and skin burns do not occur.

REFERENCES

1. Hyodo, M, Kitade, AT: **Silver Spike Point Electro Therapy,** SSP Study Group, Osaka, Japan, 1984.

2. Hussain, KK: Serum Hepatitis Associated with Repeated Acupunctures. **British Medical Journal,** 3:41-42, 1974.

3. Rogers, PAM: Serious Complications of Acupuncture...or Acupuncture Abuse. Am. **J. Acup.** 9:347-351, 1981.

4. Parwatikar, S, Brown, M, Stern, J. Ulett, GA, and Sletten, IW: Acupuncture, Hypnosis and Experiemental Pain. I. Study with Volunteers. **Acup And Electro Therapeutics Res. J.,** 3:161-190, 1978.

5. Bowsher, D: Role of the reticular Formation in Response to Noxious stimulation. **Pain,** 2:361-378, 1976 .

6. Vierck, CJ, Lineberry, CG, Lee, PK *et al*:: Prolonged Hyperalgesia Following Acupuncture in Monkeys. Life Science, 15:1277-1289, 1974.

Chapter VII

CLINICAL USES OF ACUPUNCTURE

The usefulness of acupuncture for pain relief is documented by numerous clinical reports and by theories of action that are both plausible for Western trained physicians and supported by theories concurrent with modern physiology and biochemistry. The use of acupuncture for psychosomatic illness, however, and for patients with emotional illnesses, is less well documented but has been found useful by many physicians on an empirical basis. We have obtained some surprisingly good results in the treatment of a variety of conditions that have failed to respond to more traditional medical management.

Controlled studies of acupuncture are difficult because the insertion of needles, even into non-acupuncture points, can reduce pain (1). The placebo effect alone can account for 30% of the relief. Good studies, however, have shown that acupuncture is effective in 55-85% of patients with chronic pain. Review of clinical reports worldwide (2) shows figures hovering around the 70% success rate. My own experience has included several thousand patients running the gamut from low back sprain and myalgia to radiculitis with sciatica, osteoarthritis, fibrositis, disc problems, post-herpetic neuralgia, trigeminal and atypical facial pain, headaches, sports injuries, carpal tunnel syndrome, diabetic neuropathies and other types of pain. These patients with such varied complaints have come after failure with the usual treatments Western medicine has to offer. The results have, on the whole, been most gratifying. Although increasingly referrals are from peer physicians, the majority of patients come at the suggestion of previous patients who have benefited from acupuncture treatments.

In my practice, as elsewhere, the major use of acupuncture is for the treatment of pain. Most common among the favorable responders are those who, treated on a once weekly basis, get only a small amount of relief after a treatment or two but then continue on with steady improvement week after week to a point where, with 8-10 treatments, the pain is usually controlled. At that point treatment can be given at bi-monthly or monthly intervals. Many patients who receive almost complete relief require no additional treatments. Mine is an experience from private practice and hence there is no good follow-up of patients. There have, however, been frequent reports from new patients who state that they were referred to us by former patients of ours who have continued to do well over periods of months or years. I have had many patients with arthritic and neuralgic conditions return with a pain that has resumed after an asymptomatic period of many months. They ask to again experience the relief that they experienced with the original course of treatments and often this is accomplished with fewer treatments than were required initially.

These clinical observations have served to strengthen my opinion that acupuncture acts in some "kindling like" fashion that has a cumulative effect of dampening the reverberating activity in neuron pools. Such pools have a self-sustaining activity that tends to maintain the pain threshold such that even the smallest increase in physical or emotional stress can produce suffering. With repeated stimuli from acupuncture treatments, one sees a steady, though sometimes uneven, remitting of such activity, a rise in pain threshold and, with the best of results a dropping out of pain-producing activity. Undoubtedly these "pain memory" pools exist at several levels of the central nervous system including the cerebral cortex. I have successfully treated patients with phantom limb pain whose painful memories included the exact position of the limb at the time of an accident, a position which steadily corrected itself to a normal resting position with repeated electro-acupuncture treatments.

I have treated cases of visceral pain, usually by vagal (ear) stimulation as well as posterior root stimulation at the level of visceral innervation. Results in the treatment of chronic nerve and muscle degenerative diseases, multiple sclerosis, stroke, nerve deafness and the like seem much more likely to be the result of some general subjective improvement and probably have a larger placebo component. The fact that some such patients have, when undergoing acupuncture, reported an increased tempo in their rate of improvement has encouraged me to at least offer persons with these types of illness a trial of acupuncture treatment. We have had good success with cases of tic, pre-eclampsia and spasmodic torticollis.

Acupuncture is also used for a variety of psychiatric conditions including depression, anxiety, insomnia, tension and nervousness. It has been suggested that the serotonin, enkephalin and endorphin release which occurs with acupuncture involves as well the release of growth hormone and prolactin (3, 4, 5, 6). This hormonal release gives some credence to the use of acupuncture in such a wide range of conditions. I also believe that stimulation of the concha of the ear with direct activation of the vagus nerve produces an anti-anxiety effect that is important in the treatment of many conditions.

Wen (7), reported with electro-acupuncture an induced sense of well-being and suppression of the symptoms of sympathetic hyperactivity seen upon withdrawal of opiates. Ng (8,9), of the National Institutes of Health, also reported that such ear electro-stimulation reduced the withdrawal symptoms of addiction. Others, following Wen's technique, have also reported good results with various forms of addiction. Some others reported success using treatments based upon the metaphysical concepts of auriculotherapy. Such treatments use needles only, without electrical stimulation. One well recognized group of researchers (10) using a single blind study, published significant results using such technique. They were, however, careful to place their active needles in the concha of the ear and had their control needles inserted outside of this area. Such treatments fail to take advantage of the stronger effect that could be produced by using electrical stimulation. Thus it was predictable that the results of a meta-analysis of all published controlled studies of acupuncture used for addiction has yielded negative results (11). It is my opinion that it was the electrical stimulation of the vagal area of the concha that was responsible for Wen's very significant positive results. We have found electrical stimulation to be generally more effective than needles alone and hence treat chemical dependent patients with an electrically stimulated polymer pad electrode filling the concha of the ear. I recommend this as the superior approach to patients with such illness.

Acupuncture is not a replacement for surgical anesthesia. At best it will play a very small role in Western surgery, despite the fact that it has much to offer. Electro-acupuncture produces analgesia, but not true anesthesia. Thus, the patient is aware of sensations other than pain and in some cases the pain itself is not entirely abolished, but is only reduced in intensity. While this may be of great benefit to some patients, allowing them to avoid the common complications and discomfort that occur with general anesthesia, there are risks and inconveniences that Western surgeons are loathe to assume. Relaxation is poor, especially when abdominal incisions are required. Anxious patients become even more so when placed in the strangeness of a surgical amphitheater. The procedure is more time consuming than chemical anesthesia and is limited to those patients who are good acupuncture responders.

Some 30% of patients fail to respond to acupuncture. This is approximately the same number who fail to respond to the administration of morphine (12). Like Pomeranz's rats (13), these persons possibly have some inherited defect in their opiate receptor systems. As demonstrated by Han's group, such persons may fail to have an adequate endorphin release upon acupuncture stimulation. The administration of DL-phenylalanine can convert some patients from non-responders to responders, but more work remains to be done to determine how best to help this group of patients.

Table III lists the conditions suggested by the World Health Organization as amenable to acupuncture treatment. The list was given without statistics or proof of effectiveness and is thus simply a statement of common practice in some parts of the world. There have been many reports of single or multiple cases of all of these types of illness treated with some success. Such reports appear scattered throughout the acupuncture literature, including books on traditional acupuncture and journals such as the *American Journal of Chinese Medicine* and *American Journal of Acupuncture*. Many of these reports are couched in metaphysical language, refer to traditional acupuncture theory and have no semblance of acceptable scientific standards. Others do give a comparison of results with standard medical treatment practices. The percentage of success will vary depending upon whether the cases treated are acute or chronic.

In some instances reports in the literature state that there is significant improvement in up to 90% of patients treated. These reports may well have been biased by including numerous acutely ill patients who came to acupuncture as an initial mode of treatment for illnesses that were essentially self-limited. It is generally recognized that patients with low back pain who have not had surgery do better than patients who have been operated upon.

One of the most widely circulated tabulations of the success of acupuncture treatments is found in the writings of Felix Mann (14). He compiled the treatment results of 10 doctors who reported on 1,000 patients. Forty-four percent of patients were listed as "cured or markedly improved" and 20% showed moderate improvement for a total of 64% of patients who benefited from acupuncture treatments. Mann also quotes the work of Bischko (15), including some 2,812 patients of whom 36% had "good results" and 25% who were listed as "plus minus" for a total of 61% of patients who were helped to some extent. An even larger treatment series from the Washington, D.C. Acupuncture Center (16) reported 80% of 11,982 patients having significant improvement. However, the author states that the methods for collection of this information were "not entirely objective and scientific."

The National Institute of Health's special ad hoc committee met to consider the many suggested uses of acupuncture. As reported by Howard Jenerick (17); "clinical investigators at eight separate pain clinics reported on acupuncture versus placebo treatments of acute and chronic pain in over 400 patients. Individual complaints and diagnoses ranged over a wide spectrum including phantom limb pain, causalgia and other neuropathy, headache and migraine, rheumatoid and osteoarthritic pain, musculo-skeletal pain, etc. In many instances the patients had experienced failure with conventional treatments and had been referred to the pain clinic by their original attending physician. On the order of 60% of all patients reported good to excellent relief from their pain for periods ranging from hours to months. Results varied according to the underlying pathology. The best outcome was obtained with self-limiting diseases, although some conditions of long standing (i.e., chronic headache, arthritis, low back pain) also responded well."

TABLE III
MEDICAL CONDITIONS
FOR WHICH ACUPUNCTURE IS COMMONLY USED.

Bronchitis and asthma	Conjunctivitis
Coronary heart disease	Acute and chronic rhinitis
Hypertension	Acute tonsillitis
Peptic ulcer	Arthritis
Disease of biliary tract	Shoulder pain
Acute and chronic gastritis	Neck strain
Dysmenorrhea	Tenosynovitis
Morning sickness	Headache
Acute simple appendicitis	Acute and chronic lumbago
Urticaria	Sciatica
Neurasthenia	Facial nerve paralysis
Enuresis	Toothache
Vertigo	Acute sprains
Sequelae of Cerebro-vascular accidents	Intercostal neuralgia and herpes Zoster

From: Bannerman, RH.: The World Health Organization's Viewpoint on Acupuncture. *Amer. J. Acupuncture.* 8:231-236, 1980.

Matsumoto, Professor of Surgery and Director of Surgical Research at Hahnemann Medical college, Philadelphia, conducted single and double blind studies of the efficacy of acupuncture in the treatment of chronic neck and shoulder pain due to osteoarthritis (18). He concluded that acupuncture was effective and that there was a statistically significant difference between the patients who received acupuncture at specific points and those who were stimulated at non-specific points. Those patients who had had previous surgery for low back pain tended to do less well with acupuncture. Back pain is one of the most common afflictions of the human race. Patients with this complaint will make up the bulk of any acupuncturist's practice. I have found electro-acupuncture to be an effective treatment for many of these patients (19).

Mendelson (20) reviewed published reports on the use of acupuncture in the treatment of chronic pain. He looked at both controlled and uncontrolled studies. Among 765 patients in six uncontrolled clinical reports, there was a 70% improvement reported. In six controlled studies involving 417 patients, the reports showed equal success with either placebo or acupuncture in four studies, and a significantly higher percentage with acupuncture in two of the studies. Mendelson felt that there are few studies of acupuncture that meet high standards for validity. Nonetheless he stated that "...on balance of evidence it appears that acupuncture has a place in the management of chronic pain resistant to orthodox treatment measures." The previously cited meta-analysis (11) agrees with Mendelson that there are few well controlled studies in the literature. They conclude that acupuncture is little more than placebo. Such discrepancies could well occur from the fact that there is little uniformity of treatment techniques, and that the placement of needles is usually based on nebulous metaphysical concepts. Electrical stimulation is not always used and when it is used the parameters of stimulation are often not adequately reported. More definitive answers can be given when acupuncturists use more uniform electro-acupuncture techniques and discard metaphysical theories about acupuncture in favor of methods based upon known scientific facts.

It is my own conclusion that acupuncture has a markedly analgesic effect as demonstrated by its use for surgery which I have witnessed in China. Most writers on this subject tend to stress either the "physical" or "psychological" as being responsible for the analgesic effect. It is, however, now apparent that any comprehensive theory of acupuncture analgesia will have to consider a possible combined effect of both physiological and psychological mechanisms.

In summary, it would appear that acupuncture is best used for the treatment of various types of pain, both acute and chronic. For such conditions the clinical results will often be very good. Usually both physiological and psychological factors will be at work. Acupuncture is often the treatment of choice for pain conditions. Here it has a chance of producing some lasting relief as compared to the short term effect of pain suppressing analgesics. These latter also invariably show a propensity for side effects and addiction which are not present with acupuncture. For other non-pain conditions, acupuncture should be reserved for only those illnesses that do not respond favorably with Western type treatment methods.

It is essential that the decision to treat patients by acupuncture be made by medically trained persons who are in a position to determine whether the condition considered for treatment is indeed suitable for acupuncture or whether some other type of treatment might be more appropriate and effective. This is especially true in serious illnesses where more conventional type of treatment needs to be rapidly instituted to save life or to prevent additional suffering that might develop with the delay occasioned were reliance placed solely upon acupuncture. Often electro-acupuncture can be effectively used in combination with some other types of treatment for the best results. In the final analysis electro-acupuncture is but one of many medical treatments from among which the physician may select. When used properly it can significantly add to the therapeutic armamentarium.

References

1. Parwatikar, S., Brown, M., Stern, J., Ulett, G.: Acupuncture, Hypnosis and Experimental Pain. I, Study with Volunteers. **Acup and Electro-Therapeutics Res. J.** 3:161-90, 1978.

2. Lu, Gwei-Djen and Needham, J.: **Celestial Lancets** Cambridge University Press, p. 427, 1980.

3. Shaar, CJ., Frederickson, RCA., and Dininger, NB. et al: Enkephalin Analogues and Naloxone by an Endogenous Opioid Peptide in Brain. **Life Science** 21:853-860, 1977.

4. Cocchi, D., Santagostino, A., Gil-Ad, I., *et al.*: Leu-enkephalin-stimulated growth hormone with Prolactin Release in the Rat: Comparison with the Effect of Morphine. **Life Science,** 20:2041-2045, 1977.

5. Dupont, A., Cusan, L., Garon, M., *et al.:* Beta-endorphin Stimulation of Growth Hormone Release in Vivo. **Proc. Natl. Acad. Sci.**, USA 74:358-359, 1977.

6. River, C., Vale, W., Ling, N., *et al.:* Stimulation in vivo of the secretion of Prolactin and Growth Hormone by B-Endorphin. **Endocrinol. 100: 238-241, 1977.**

7. Wen, HC. and Teo, SW.: Experience in the treatment of Drug Addiction by electro-acupuncture. *Mod. Med. Asia.* 11:23-24, 1975.

8. Ng, LKY., Douthitt, TC., Thoa, NB., *et al.:* Modification of morphine withdrawal syndrome in rats following transauricular electrostimulation: an experimental paradigm for auricular electroacupuncture. **Biol. Psychiat** 10:575-580, 1975.

9. Ng, LKY: *Acupuncture in the Management of Narcotic Dependency.* A Presentation of Acupuncture. Connecticut State Medical Society, Farmington, Conn. September 29, 1975.

10. Lipton, DS., Brewington, V. and Smith, M.: *Acupuncture and Crack Addicts. A Single-Blind Placebo Test of Efficacy.* Presented at the NIDA Technical review Meeting, advances in Cocaine treatment, August 16-17, 1990.

11. Ter Riet, G., Kleijnen, J., Knipschild, P.: Acupuncture and chronic pain: a criteria-based meta-analysis. *J. Clin. Epidemiol,* 43: 1191-1199, 1990.

12. Beecher, HK.,: Placebo analgesia in human volunteers. **JAMA** 159: 1602-1606, 1955.

13. Peets, J. and Pomeranz, B.: CXBX mice deficient in opiate receptors show poor electro-acupuncture analgesia. *Nature* 273:675-676, 1978.

14. Mann, F.: **Scientific Aspects of Acupuncture,** William Heinemann Medical Books, Ltd, London, p. 77. 1977.

15. Bischko, J.: From the Vienna Allgemaine Poliklinic as reported by Felix Mann In, **Acupuncture, the Ancient Chinese Art of Healing and How It Works Scientifically.** Vintage Books, 1973.

16. **Wensel, LO.: Acupuncture in Medical Practice.** Reston Publishing Co. p. 333, 1980.

17. Jenerick, HP.: The NIH Acupuncture Research Study. As reported in Warren, FZ.: **Handbook of Medical Acupuncture.** Von Nostrand Reinhold Company. p. 273, 1976.

18. Matsumoto, T: **Acupuncture for Physicians.** C.C. Thomas, Springfield, IL. p. 204, 1974.

19. Ulett, GA. Acupuncture. In. Tollison, CD and Kriegel ML (eds.) *Rehabilitation of Low Back Pain. A Nonsurgical Approach.* Williams and Wilkins, Baltimore, 1989.

20. Mendelson, G.: Acupuncture Analgesia, II Review of Current Theories. **Aust. N.Z. J., Med.** 8:100-105, 1978.

Chapter VIII

LEGAL CONSIDERATIONS

In many parts of the world it is accepted that acupuncture is effective for pain relief and some other conditions. Now that sufficient scientific, clinical and experimental evidence exists to replace fanciful Yin and Yang explanations with acceptable medical knowledge, why is acupuncture not embraced wholeheartedly by Western medicine?

First of all, acupuncture was thrust into Western prominence in an unfavorable manner. Most medical innovations come from laboratory experiments and are given some prolonged preliminary testing and evaluation, both at the animal and clinical level. They are then announced to the public press, via scientists, physicians and medical schools. Acupuncture had no such introduction. It had its origin in folk medicine, shrouded in centuries of Oriental mysticism, numerology and metaphysics. It was brought to public attention in the United States by the news media with great fanfare. It caught the public fancy and was widely touted as a medical miracle and cure-all before the medical profession was aware of its full implications as a method of treatment. A demand for acupuncture rapidly developed throughout the Western world, yet there was no place that physicians could readily acquire scientifically based knowledge and training. Available books were simply translations of centuries old mystical beliefs of alterations in some mysterious body energy not mentioned in medical school. To practice such a mumbo jumbo ritual was anathema to scientifically trained physicians.

Shortly, after its reintroduction into the United States there began to appear reports of experimental work from the People's Republic of China and elsewhere. These strongly indicated mechanisms within the central nervous system which offered scientifically acceptable theories and results of experiments upon acupuncture's action for pain relief. These theories were just as conclusive as the theoretical basis of many treatments used in medical practice today. Such scientific evidence could well have justified the inclusion of acupuncture within

112

the physicians' armamentarium but, given the skeptical attitude of their peers, only a few brave physicians ventured into this field. The official stand of American medicine remained a negative one.

With lifting of the "bamboo curtain," some physicians toured China to see for themselves acupuncture in its native setting, Many were unable to explain what they saw and labeled acupuncture as some form of Chinese stoicism or hypnotic induction. The public interest and demand to try this new "cure-all" treatment continued to grow. Fringe medical groups soon sensed a golden opportunity. Acupuncture clinics were established, some staffed by acupuncture technicians imported from the Orient and acting under the umbrella of licensed physicians. Chinese herb doctors, long practicing unnoticed in the Chinatowns of New York, San Francisco and elsewhere, enjoyed a new found legitimacy. At this time there was growing public dissatisfaction with Western medicine. This opened the door for "holistic" and "alternative therapists" who, without medical knowledge and feeling no necessity to adopt forms of treatment based on scientific facts, simply opened shop as "doctors of acupuncture."

Skepticism concerning a new (or recently re-introduced) treatment is characteristic of the medical profession while just the opposite appears to be the case with non-medically trained laymen and cultic health practitioners. In all peoples throughout the world there has always been a strong belief in mysticism and the occult. Such belief is strengthened by the hope and desire to find some miracle remedy to relieve pain and chronic suffering. This is especially true when these symptoms have not responded well to the usual medical remedies. "Why not," they say, "try this new cure-all acupuncture?"

It was probably this spectre of quackery that moved the AMA to expel acupuncture from their grace of approval and in July, 1981, the House of Delegates of the American Medical Association took a stand, calling acupuncture an "unproven modality of therapy" (1). This pronouncement by the AMA, which was taken to protect the public from unproven therapies, may actually have served to further promote the use of acupuncture by persons without proper medical training. If patients could not get the treatment from their family physician they would seek it elsewhere.

I emphasized this possibility when I appeared before the 1975 Annual Meeting of the Federation of State Medical Boards (2). This warning went unheeded however and by 1991 22 states had issued licenses to non-medical persons for the unsupervised practice of acupuncture. Requirements for certification vary from 50 to 500 hours of training in what amounts to an exercise in Oriental metaphysics. It is an anachronism that M.D.'s and D.O.'s, whose license permits them to do surgery and intravenous procedures, must also take several hundred hours of Oriental metaphysics in order to be permitted to perform the simple maneuvers spelled out in this book. Such treatment procedures require only the knowledge already acquired in medical school plus a minimal amount of instruction.

There is continuing strong pressure by non-medical lobbying groups for acupuncture certification in all 50 states, for recognition of acupuncture needles and apparatus by the FDA and for payment by Medicare and third party payers for the practice of acupuncture. Regarding the latter, there is much confusion as most insurance companies do not pay for acupuncture. Others do, and some only when it is called by such names as neuro-electric stimulation. Some pay when the procedure is done by an M.D. or D.O. and others when it is performed by a non-medical acupuncturist with state certification. It is of interest that many insurers will pay for TENS treatments and apparatus apparently not recognizing that such treatments are in reality electro-acupuncture.

Most non-medical acupuncturists practice traditional acupuncture and are associated with and call themselves practitioners of Traditional Chinese Medicine. As pointed out in this text there is now sufficient grounds to distinguish physiological or scientific acupuncture from the traditional or metaphysical variety. Much confusion might thus be avoided if a distinction for licensing were to be made between practitioners of Traditional Chinese Medicine including the metaphysical variety of acupuncture and those who use Western methods of diagnosis and physiologically based electro-acupuncture or neuro-electric stimulation. The latter could be readily subsumed under existing licenses for the practice of medicine without the need for additional certification.

A report from the Hastings Center in April of 1981 (3) referred to a ruling by a Federal Court Judge in Texas who stated that the Texas Medical Practice Act to limit the practice of acupuncture to duly licensed physicians was an unconstitutional invasion of the individual's right to seek the treatment of his/her choice. This Texas statute that was so weakened, is typical of statutes that exist in other states to protect citizens from the sale of quack cancer cures and other types of charlatanism. The reasoning behind this Texas action demonstrates the woeful lack of knowledge about acupuncture existing among legal, legislative and regulatory board members. Such groups fail to distinguish between metaphysics and science. They thus ignore the advances in medicine made over the last 3000 years and support the licensure of persons who lack the training necessary to properly diagnose the illnesses they propose to treat. This creates the possibility of an improper treatment being used for conditions which might well require an approach other than acupuncture. Such a failure poses a danger to health and life.

An additional problem faced by the physician who plans to treat by acupuncture is the FDA's regulation concerning the equipment used for such treatments. Electronic stimulators and needles used in acupuncture must still be labeled as "experimental devices." This may present a problem for physicians who wish to import treatment apparatus such as that available from sources in the Orient.

Another consideration is the question of malpractice insurance. Special policies are now available for persons practicing acupuncture. These usually require that the person seeking coverage be certified or licensed to do acupuncture by the state in which he/she practices. If the person is practicing neuroelectric treatment based upon scientific medical principles or using a TENS stimulator, it would be presumed that no such special malpractice coverage need be obtained. However, because these treatments are usually conceived as being "acupuncture" in nature, the company issuing the malpractice insurance may very well request an additional premium. In the opinion of William Dornette, M.D., Director of Education and Research, Division of Anesthesiology at the Cleveland Clinic in Cleveland, Ohio (4), "...the use of this technique by a licensed practitioner who has had training in acupuncture and has a thorough knowledge in anatomy poses no more, and certainly far less, risk to the patient than many other therapeutic modalities."

With the widespread use of disposable needles the risk of acupuncture to the patient is practically nil. It is always wise however to have some type of informed consent. It may be sufficient to furnish the patient with a description of acupuncture and its possible side effects or the patient may sign a release form indicating that acupuncture is still considered an "experimental" form of treatment. We have recently developed a three minute video tape that explains the procedure and risks to the patient in graphic form. This is an excellent way to explain and reassure the patient. It also would clearly explain to any court of law exactly what understanding the patient had about the procedure used.

REFERENCES

1. AMA Council of Scientific Affairs. **Reports of the Council on Scientific Affairs of the American Medical Association, Chicago, 1981.** American Medical Association, 1982.

2. Ulett, GA.: Acupuncture – A Technique for the Regularly Licensed Physician. **Federal Bulletin.** 62:334-343, 1975.

3. Schwartz, R.: Yin, Yang and the Right to Privacy. Acupuncture and Expertise. A Challenge to Physician Control. **The Hastings Center Report,** pp. 5-7, April 1981.

4. Dornette, WHL.: Acupuncture and the Law. In Warren, FX., **Handbook of Medical Acupuncture.** Van Norstrand Reinhold Co., N.Y. 1976.

Chapter IX

SPECULATION: PLACEBOS, MIND-BODY RELATIONSHIPS, ACUPUNCTURE AND CONDITIONED HEALING.

PLACEBO: The question has been asked, "Is acupuncture a placebo?" The answer is "yes, and so is every other form of treatment." For, in addition to whatever biochemical or other action any medical treatment causes in the body, there is, in addition, a strong possibility that there will also be a physiologically manifested placebo response triggered by an emotional reaction initiated in the right hemisphere.

The word **placebo** comes from the Greek meaning, "I shall please." Surely, when the treatment is successful, both patient and doctor are pleased. For the patient, placebo means "I believe," because when the patient has faith in the doctor and treatment, the placebo response is strengthened. The physician's strong belief that the treatment will be effective may be communicated to the patient verbally and also non-verbally by an air of confidence.

Although it is usually estimated that placebo response occurs in 30% of instances, in some situations it has been reported to account for an even greater amount of the treatment result. Acupuncture is a strong placebo widely believed to cure all manner of ailments. It came from the mysterious Orient. Its mode of action has long been a mystery cloaked in magical terms. Needles themselves have a mystique all of their own.

In those long dark years prior to the 19th Century, medicine had little to offer but placebo treatment, hope, support and magic rituals. The administration of cupping, purging, plasters and cathartics added little to the curative effect of placebo. Today we are so accustomed to thinking of medicine in scientific terms that we forget that for thousands of years patients were cured by witch doctors and charlatans with little scientific or medical knowledge. Acupuncture was born in those dark days and has, along with other folk medicines, come to us shrouded in superstition and metaphysical explanations. Its placebo strength has kept it alive through the centuries. Despite the fact that acupuncture has been found to have a scientific basis, it still retains the power of placebo.

Today, for reasons of custom, ignorance or design, thousands of acupuncturists practice ancient metaphysical forms of acupuncture and simply place needles in various body loci as determined by pulse diagnosis, or some equally mystical, arcane formula. Such practices continue despite evidence that only a few of the thousand acupuncture points have any physiological effect, that electrical stimulation is essential for maximal effect and that acupuncture is really frequency specific and not point specific. Thus many acupuncturists today are actually practicing *Placebo Acupuncture.*

Early studies showed that the pain reducing effect of the placebo can be blocked by giving the drug naloxone. Naloxone blocks the effect of morphine and opioid hormones. Thus, from these preliminary experiments it was hypothesized that the placebo produces its effect through the release of endorphins. The placebo appears to act in the same manner as acupuncture through an effect on brain neuropeptides.

From the evidence given in this book, it is clear that when electrical stimulation is added, acupuncture becomes a "real" treatment. This may add significantly to its already existing placebo strength. The placebo has been, and remains, a powerful weapon in the physician's therapeutic arsenal. Its potency is demonstrated by the fact that quacks, using only placebos, are often as effective as physicians using scientific methods.

MIND-BODY INTERACTIONS   The interrelationship between mind and body, is being explored in laboratories around the world. The new name for the study of this ancient concept is *Psycho-immunology.* Since 1976 there have been nearly 2000 references in the literature on this subject.

Although it is still too early to describe with certainty the manner in which behavior promotes illness or healing, we can say that there is now clear and irrefutable evidence that the central nervous system and the immune system communicate regularly. Somewhere in the distant phylogeny the immune system was part of the brain. Immune cells have developed receptors for neurotransmitters and neuropeptides. One fundamental characteristic of cells of both the nervous and the immune system is the capacity for memory. In sensitized lymphocytes there is the memory that permits the antigen antibody reaction. In the brain memory is necessary for life, and according to Melzack it may well be the basis for chronic pain.

Certain combinations of stressors and buffers in the social environment, coupled with the personal characteristics of an individual, determine the way in which a person perceives a stressor and subsequently adapts psychologically.

Maladaptive behavior, as measured by symptoms of insomnia, anxiety or depression for example, is then postulated to mediate changes in neuroendocrine and autonomic efferent pathways from the brain altering immune function and affecting disease susceptibility and health outcome. The death of a spouse, melancholia, the stress of examinations, and the strain of care giving have all been demonstrated to produce immune dysfunction.

In contrast, stress-management interventions such as relaxation, anxiety reduction and social support have all been found to improve immune functions. Good evidence exists from several laboratories that an increase in serum concentration of endogenous opioids, including metenkephalin, Beta-lipotropin and Beta-endorphin, have direct effects on immunity. A focus of current interest is the demonstrated effect of psychologically induced changes creating a more severe stage of the immuno-deficiency reaction in subjects with early HIV infection. On the other hand, psychological factors that tend to moderate the progress of this disease include those that are known to reduce stress.

The above paragraph gives some rational for the increasing number of clinical reports stating that acupuncture is of some benefit in cases of disorders of the immune system, including asthma, eczema and more recently, in persons suffering from AIDS. If, indeed, traditional acupuncture has any positive effect on disease as a result of its powerful placebo action, it could be even more beneficial to use the greater stimulating action of electro-acupuncture. Thus we can add the prefix "neuro" and investigations of this type of treatment phenomenon could be rightly subsumed under the term, *neuro-psycho-immunology*, and this method of treatment might be called *neuro-psycho-acupuncture*.

CONDITIONED HEALING Another intriguing method of using electro-acupuncture involves training patients to self stimulate the release of neuropeptides. This possibility is suggested by a series of landmark experiments described by Robert Ader (1) and his colleagues who showed that the immune response in experimental animals could be classically conditioned. Watkins, et al. (2), induced analgesia in rats by neuroelectrical stimulation of the front paws. When the electrical stimulation was paired with a tone in repeated experiments, it later became possible to produce analgesia by presenting the tone alone. This has been termed, "auto-analgesia" (3). The same thing happened when animals were merely put into the cage where the conditioning had occurred. This response could be blocked by nalorphine, thus demonstrating that opioids were involved in what could be more properly termed a conditioned analgesic phenomenon.

It would be possible to set up a classical conditioning paradigm in human subjects to teach them to self release neural peptides including among them, enkephalins, endorphins and ACTH.

Rather than using a tone or bell for conditioning stimulus it would be preferable in humans to use a mental image which would always be conveniently available. Unlike a tone (an external conditioning signal), images are electrochemical events which are already internally woven into the fabric of the brain (4).

Imagery has always played a key role in medicine and of itself could have some therapeutic significance that would be strengthened by the electroacupuncture stimulation. Clinically, imagery has been used to stimulate the body in such a way as to strengthen the immune system (5,6).

Enkephalins and endorphins are important in imagery. The placebo effect is a dramatic example of imagination in action, a mechanism mediated by endorphins (7,8). Endorphins are formed in the anterior pituitary gland and in opioid neurons in the brain as part of a precursor, pro-opio-melano-cortin (8). On activation this precursor releases endogenous opioids and adrenocorticotropin (ACTH) (9) Enkephalins are endogenous immunomodulators). This relationship of endorphins to the immune system and of Beta-endorphin to the imagination suggests these compounds play a role in healing. Accessing this system by a combined imagery-conditioning electro-stimulation approach should provide a particularly strong signal for neuro-peptide release and thus be of considerable significance in treating disease.

Even if the image is only a small part of the total experience, it can, according to Pribram's holographic model of brain functioning (10), recreate much of the positive experience and affect of the original situation. With this in mind, we have recently been having patients self select a relaxing scene from their past experiences. A relaxation tape is used to induce a state of relaxation and self-hypnosis during which the patient images the scene that will become the conditioning stimulus. This pairing occurs during a 30-minute period of electroacupuncture in which the stimulus frequency is varied, thus releasing both endorphins and dynorphins and possibly other healing neuropeptides. This procedure is repeated over a period of several weeks. In between treatments the patient is directed to practice at home, three or more times a day, sitting quietly and visualizing the conditioning scene. In this manner he/she presumably learns to self-release neuropeptides that may be helpful in regulating the body's homeostatic mechanisms.

The above discourse suggests ways in which acupuncture might be integrated into treatment programs not only for pain, but also other conditions. I am sure that in the future many other ways will emerge for acupuncture to be usefully integrated into modern medical practice. Like the proverbial Phoenix of Chinese mythology, such new scientific methods for the use of electro-acupuncture will arise from the metaphysical ashes of traditional acupuncture theory and practice.

REFERENCES

1. Ader, R. and Cohen, V: Behaviorally conditioned immunosuppression and murine systemic lupus erythematosus. *Science* 215:1534-36, 1982.

2. Watkins, LR. Cobelli, AD and Mayer DJ.: Classical conditioning of front paw and hind paw footshock-induced analgesia (FSIA): Naloxone reversibility and descending pathways. *Brain Research,* 243: 119-132. 1982.

3. Chance, WT.: Autoanalgesia: Opiate and non-opiate mechanisms. *Neuroscience Biobehavioral Review,* 4:55-67, 1979.

4. Achterberg, J.: *Imagery in Healing.* New Science Library: Boston, MA, 1985.

5. Loh, YP. and Loriaux, LL.: Adrenocorticotropic hormone, P-lipotropin, and endorphin-related peptides in health and disease. *JAMA,* 247:1033-1034, 1982.

6. Swaab, DR., Achterberg, PH., Boer, BJ., Dogterom, J. and Van Leeuwen, FW.: The distribution of MSHG and ACTH in the rat and human brain and its relation to pituitary stores. In J.L. Martinex et al. (Eds.) *Endogenous Peptides and Learning Memory Processes.* Academic Press: New York, NY. 7-36, 1981.

7. Levine, JD., Godron, NC., and Fields, HL: The mechanism of placebo analgesia. *The Lancet,* Sept. 23, 654-657, 1978.

8. Kaada, B.: Is the mystery of the placebo effect about to be solved: A Pavlovian reflex for activating self-healing mechanisms. In Roilv Gjessing and Arne Graven, (Eds.) *In commemoration of the centenary of his birth.* Kikemark Hospital Press, Oslo, 43-61, 1987.

9. Niuwenhuys, R.: *Chemoarchitecture of the brain.* Springer Verlag: Berlin, 1985.

10. Pribram, K. *Language of the Brain,* Monteray CA: Brooks/Cole Pub. Co., 1971.

Appendix

SEVENTY-FIVE USEFUL POINTS FOR ACUPUNCTURE TREATMENT

Tables showing point location on regions of the body with abbreviations, anatomical location and physiological justification for point use.

Figures illustrating similarity of point location between motor points and traditional Chinese acupuncture points.

Diagrams showing motor point locations on major muscles of the body.

SEVENTY-FIVE USEFUL POINTS FOR ACUPUNCTURE TREATMENT

HEAD

Region	Name	Anatomical Location	Physiologic Justification
Vertex	VG-20	Bisection of sagittal line with line joining tragi	Supraorbital n. meets C^2C^3
Temporal	EM-1	At midpoint of a line one fingerbreath to lateral end of eyebrow and outer canthus of eye	Auriculo temporal n. Deep temporal br. of V n.
Supra-Orbital	BL-2	Above supraorbital notch	Corrugator motor point. Supra-orbital br. of V n. Temporal and infraorbital n. of VII n.
Mid-Infra-Orbital	ST-1	Just above inferior orbital region	Orbicularis oculi motor point. Infraorbital br. of V n. Facial n.
Median Canthus	BL-1	Just above median canthus	Infratrochlear n. of V
Inferior Masseter	ST-6	Junction of upper 2/3 to lower 1/3 of Masseter	Masseter motor point of V
Anterior Mastoid	TH-17	Posterior to the lobule of the auricle and in the depression between the mastoid process and the ramus of the mandible.	Lesser occipital n. C^2C^3 Greater auricular n. C^2C^3
Mandibular	TH-21	With mouth open, temporo-mandibular joint	Auriculo temporal n. Facial n.
Nasolabial Fold	LI-20	Nasolabial fold within the fold of cheek at level of interior edge of ala nasi	Infraorbital br. of V. Buccal br. of VII
Infra-Nasal	GB-26	Midline in the orbicularis oris, 2/3 superior to the margin of upper lip	Infraorbital br. of V. Zygomatic br. of VII
Anterior Tragus	SI-19	In front of the tragus at the depression made when the mouth is slightly open	Auriculo temporal br. of V. Facial n.
Lateral Oral Angle	ST-4	1/2 cm lateral to angle of mouth	Orbicularis oris motor point mental n. Cervico facial br. of VII n.
Antero-Lateral Mandible	ST-5	Inferior edge of mandible anterior to the gonion, lower anterior border of masseter muscle	Buccal ramus of facial nerve
Anterior Ear	ST-7	Under the zygomatic arch in front of the condyle of the mandible. In the hollow that fills upon opening the jaw	Branches of the temporal and internal pterygoid nerves

NECK

Region	Name	Anatomical Location	Physiologic Justification
Sub-occipital	GB-20	Just lateral to trapezius at occiput	Greater occipital C_2 posterior primary ramus
Supraspinous Ligament	GV-15	Supraspinous ligament between C_1 - C_2 spinous process midline	Posterior ramus C_2 meets C_3
Paracricoid	ST-9	Anterior border of sterno-mastoid at level of cricoid	Cervical br. of facial n. anterior cutaneous C_2, C_3
Supra-Sternal	CV-22	Neck extended just above sternal notch	Anterior cutaneous n. of neck C_2, C_3
Supra-Spinous Ligament C_7- D_1	GV-14	In the supraspinal ligament, flex head just below C_7 (most prominent spinous process)	Posterior ramus C_3 meets C_4
Sterno-Cleido Mastoid	LI-18	Two fingerbreaths lateral to the mid-point of the laryngeal prominence and between the two heads of the sternocleido-mastoid muscle	Spinal accessory n. (motor) C_2, C_3 (sensory)

UPPER EXTREMITY

Region	Name	Anatomical Location	Physiologic Justification
First Dorsal Space	LI-4	1st dorsal interosseous	1st dorsal interosseous motor point
4th Dorsal Space	TH-3	Between 4-5 metacarpals	4th dorsal interosseous motor point
5th Lateral Metacarpal	SI-3	Ulnar border of and at distal palmar crease (clenched fist)	Abductor digiti quinti motor point
Dorsal Distal Forearm	TH-5	3cm proximal to distal end of radius and ulna	Extensor pollicis longus motor point
Dorsal Upper Forearm	TH-9	10cm distal to olecranon	Extensor carpi ulnaris motor point
Lateral Cubital Crease	LI-11	With elbow flexed, at lateral cubital crease	Brachioradialis motor point
Volar Distal Forearm	PC-6	3 cm proximal to proximal crease over median nerve	Median nerve
Acromio-Clavicula Joint	LI-16	Acromioclavicular joint	Supraclavicular n. (C_4)
Posterior Acromion	TH-14	Posterior aspect of acromion	Supraclavicular n. ($C_{3,4}$)
Posterior Axillary Crease	SI-9	Apex of posterior axillary fold	$D_2 D_3$ meets circulflex n. C_5, C_6
Posterior Elbow	TH-10	Posterior surface of arm, just above the point of the elbow, junction of triceps muscle with tendon	Muscle tendon junction Golgi tendon organ

Region	Name	Anatomical Location	Physiologic Justification
Radial Styloid Process	HT-7	Ulnar side of wrist on posterior border of pisiform in depression at radial side of tendon of flexor carpi ulnaris	Medial antebrachial cutaneous n. (T_1); palmar cutaneous branch of the ulnar n. (C_8, T_1); Ulnar n. (C_8, T_1)
Radial Styloid Process	LU-7	Above styloid process of radius, two fingerbreaths above transverse crease of wrist	Lateral antibrachial cutaneous ($C_{2,8}$). Superficial branch of the radial n.
Top of Shoulder	GB-21	Top of shoulder in midline between C_7 and acromion	Posterior branch of the supra-clavicular n. and branches of the cervical plexus
Upper Arm	LI-14	Lateral arm at insertion of deltoid	Auxillary n. posterior cord, posterior division upper trunk C_5C_6

CHEST AND ABDOMEN

Region	Name	Anatomical Location	Physiologic Justification
Anterior Shoulder	SP-20	Second intercostal space 8 fingerbreaths from midline	Motor point of pectoralis
Upper Lateral Arm	LU-2	Below the acromial extremity of the clavicle in the depression between deltoid and the pectoralis major	Anterior deltoid motor point
Subxiphoid	CV-15	Just below xiphoid process	D_6 and D_7 intercostal anterior cutaneous br. of anterior rami of intercostal
Inframammary	ST-18	Over 5th intercostal space at nipple line.	Obliquus externus motor point
Mid-epigastrium	CV-12	Midpoint between Xiphoid and umbilicus	D_8 and D_9 (bilateral)
Lateral Umbilicus	ST-25	Mid rectus abdominus 2 inch lateral to the umbilicus	Rectus abdominus motor point
Upper Hypogastrium	CV-6	1/5 distance between umbilicus and pubis in midline	Anterior primary ramus (bilateral) D_{11} and D_{12}
Lower Hypogastrium	CV-3	4/5 distance between umbilicus and pubis in midline	Anterior primary ramus (bilateral) D_{12} and L_1 (iliohypogastric)
Suprapubic	CV-2	Just above symphysis pubis	Anterior primary ramus (bilateral) L_1 meets S_2

LOWER EXTREMITY

Region	Name	Anatomical Location	Physiologic Justification
Posterior Trochanter	GB-30	Four fingerbreaths posterior to greater trochanter	Latreral cutaneous nerve of the thigh L_2-L_3
Midgluteal Crease	BL-50	Midline on gluteal fold	Posterior cutaneous nerve of the thigh S_3-S_4
Posterior Mid-Thigh	BL-51	Posterior mid-thigh	Posterior cutaneous nerve of the thigh S_3-S_4
Lateral Mid-Thigh	GB-31	Standing erect, where tip of long finger reaches lateral thigh	Lateral femoral cutaneous N.
Anterior Mid-Thigh	ST-32	5 fingerbreaths superior to the upper margin of patella along the line joining the lateral margin of the patella with the anterior superior iliac spine	Femoral n. posterior division lumbar plexus, L_2, L_3, L_4
Medial Supra Patella	SP-10	Three fingerbreaths above upper pole of patella over vastus medialis	Vestus femoral cutaneous n.
Medial Popliteal Crease	BL-54	Middle of popliteal fossa	Posterior femoral cutaneous n.S_2
Lateral Upper Tibialis	ST-36	Four fingerbreaths below lower pole at patella and two fingerbreaths lateral	Tibialis anterior motor point
Anterior Upper Fibula	GB-34	Neck of fibula	Peroneus longus motor point
Mid-Gastro-enemius	BL-57	Junction of medial and lateral heads of gastrocnemius in mid-calf at origin of Achilles tendon	Sural n.
Lower Tibia	SP-6	Four fingerbreaths above medial malleolus	Soleus motor point
Posterior Lateral Malleolus	BL-60	Between Achilles tendon and lateral malleolus	Flexor hallicus longus motor point
Posterior Median Malleolus	KI-3	Between Achilles tendon and medial malleolus	Superficial branch of saphenous n. L_3-L_4
Second-Third Metatarsal	ST-44	One fingerbreath proximal to web margin between second and third metatarsals	Superficial peroneal n. (L_5, S_1); Lateral plantar n. ($L_{4,5}$, $S_{1,2,3}$)
Sole of Foot	KI-1	Between second and third metatarsals on sole of foot	Medial plantar n.
Below Medial Malleolus	KI-6	Internal side of leg 2cm below the internal malleolus	Medial branches from the tibial nerve

BACK

Region	Name	Anatomical Location	Physiologic Justification
Para T_2-T_3	BL-12	Erector spinae muscles 3cm from midline para T_2-T_3	Erector spinae motor point
Para T_3-T_4	BL-13	Erector spinae muscles 3cm from midline para T_3-T_4	Erector spinae motor point
Para T_5	BL-15	One fingerbreath lateral to the inferior end of the spinous process of the 5th thoracic vertebra	Erector spinae motor point
Para T_7-T_8	BL-17	Erector spinae muscles 3cm from midline para T_7-T_8	Lower trapezius motor point
Para T_9-T_{10}	BL-18	Erector spinae muscles 3 cm from midline para T_9-T_{10}	Lower trapezius motor point
Para T_{10}-T_{11}	BL-19	Erector spinae muscles 3 cm from midline para T_{10}-T_{11}	Lower trapezius motor point
Para T_{11}-T_{12}	BL-20	Erector spinae muscles 3cm from midline para T_{11}-T_{12}	Lower trapezius motor point
Para T_{12}-L_1	BL-21	Erector spinae muscles 3cm from midline para T_{12}-L_1	Lower trapezius motor point
Para L_2-L_3	BL-23	Erector spinae muscles 3cm from midline para L_2-L_3	Lower trapezius motor point
Para L_4-L_5	BL-25	Erector spinae muscles 3cm from midline para L_4-L_5	Erector spinae motor point
Para L_5-S_1	BL-26	Erector spinae muscles 3cm from midline para L_5-S_1	Erector spinae motor point
Para S_1-S_2	BL-27	Erector spinae muscles 3cm from midline para S_1-S_2	Erector spinae motor point
Para S_2-S_3	BL-28	Erector spinae muscles 3cm from midline para S_2-S_3	Erector spinae motor point
Mid-Back	BL-40	Between sixth and seventh thoracic vertebrae three inches from midline	Trapezius motor point
Sacral Region	BL-49	Level of fourth sacral foramen three inches from midline	Gluteus maximus motor point

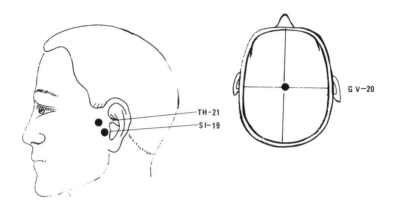

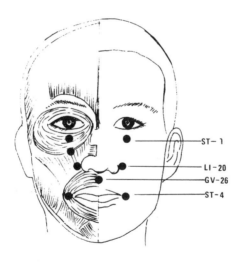

A-X: Seventy five useful acupuncture points with some corresponding or nearby motor points.*
(*After Delagi, E.F., and Perotto, A.: *Anatomic Guide for the Electromyographer.* Charles C
Thomas, Springfield, Ill., 1980.)

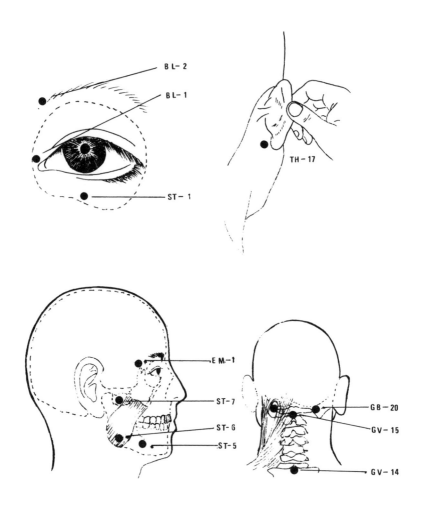

B

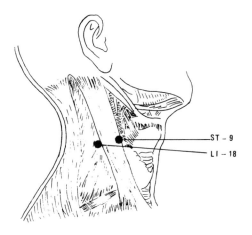

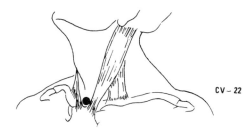

C

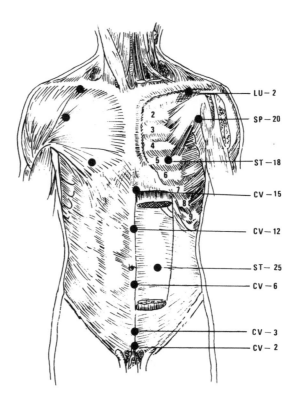

D

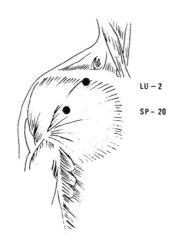

LU – 2

SP – 20

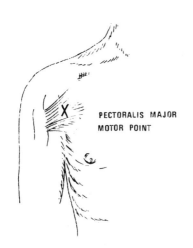

PECTORALIS MAJOR
MOTOR POINT

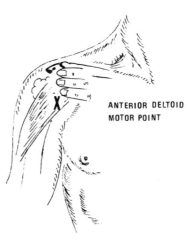

ANTERIOR DELTOID
MOTOR POINT

E

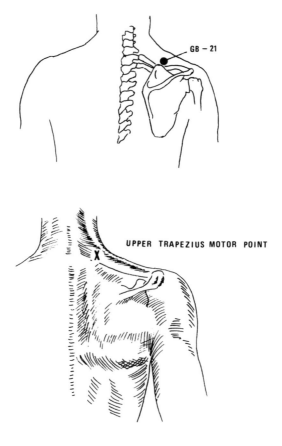

GB – 21

UPPER TRAPEZIUS MOTOR POINT

F

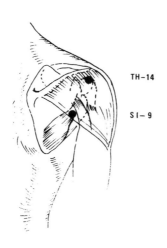

TH-14

SI-9

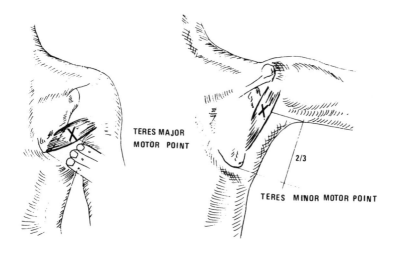

TERES MAJOR
MOTOR POINT

2/3

TERES MINOR MOTOR POINT

G

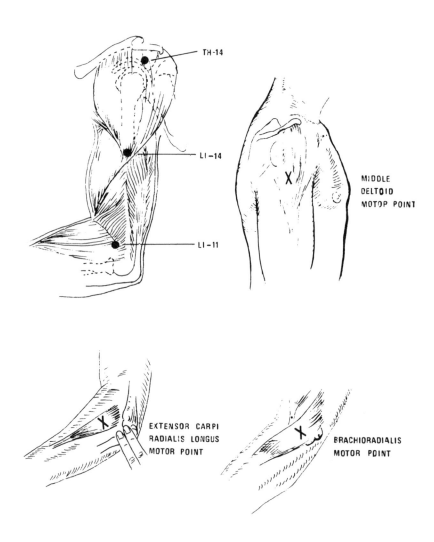

TH-14

LI-14

LI-11

MIDDLE
DELTOID
MOTOP POINT

EXTENSOR CARPI
RADIALIS LONGUS
MOTOR POINT

BRACHIORADIALIS
MOTOR PDINT

H

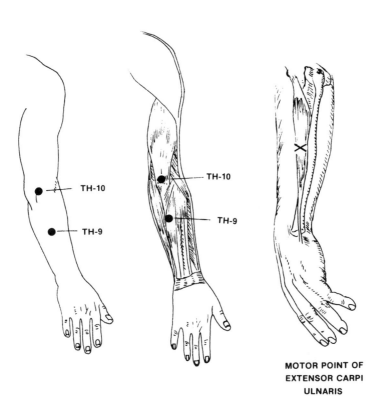

TH-10

TH-9

TH-10

TH-9

**MOTOR POINT OF
EXTENSOR CARPI
ULNARIS**

I

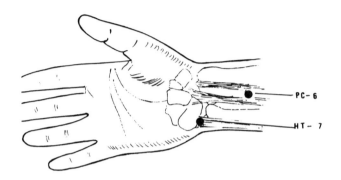

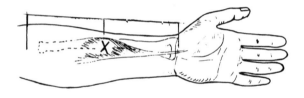

FLEXOR POLLICIS LONGUS MOTOR POINT

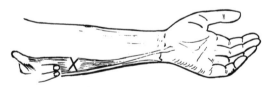

FLEXOR CARPI ULNARIS MOTOR POINT

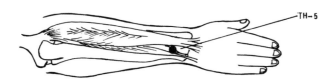

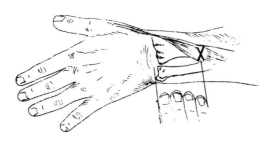

EXTENSOR POLLICIS BREVIS MOTOR POINT

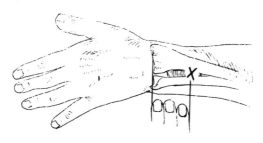

PRONATOR QUADRATUS MOTOR POINT

K

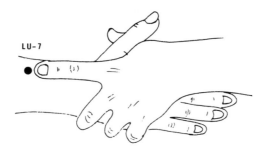

LU-7

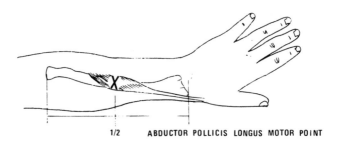

1/2   ABDUCTOR POLLICIS LONGUS MOTOR POINT

L

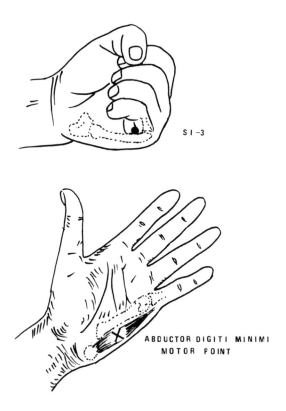

S I –3

ABDUCTOR DIGITI MINIMI
MOTOR POINT

M

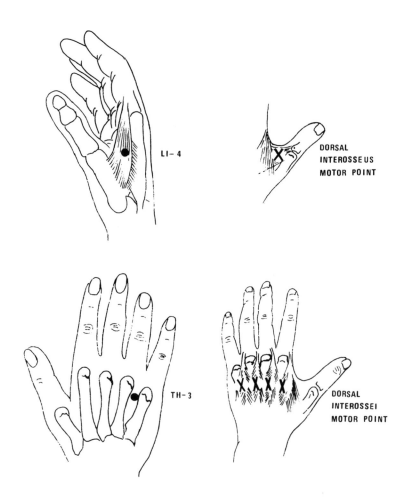

LI-4

DORSAL
INTEROSSEUS
MOTOR POINT

TH-3

DORSAL
INTEROSSEI
MOTOR POINT

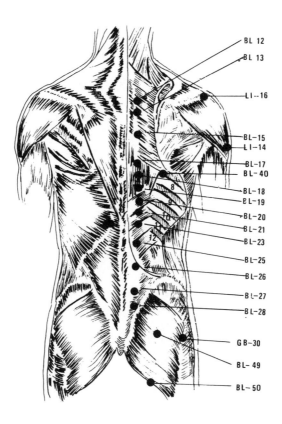

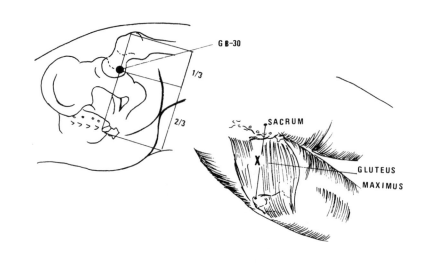

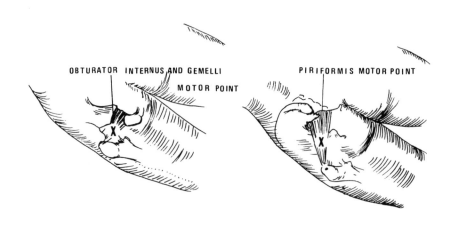

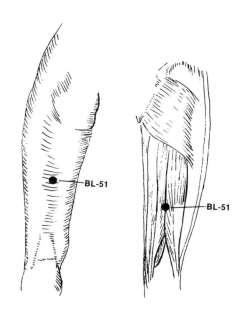

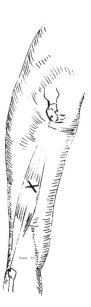

**MOTOR POINT OF
BICEPS FEMORIS
(LONG HEAD)**

Q

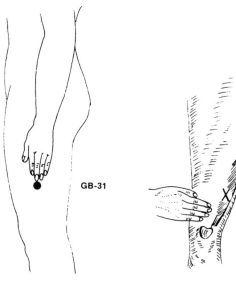

GB-31

**MOTOR POINT OF
VASTUS LATERALIS**

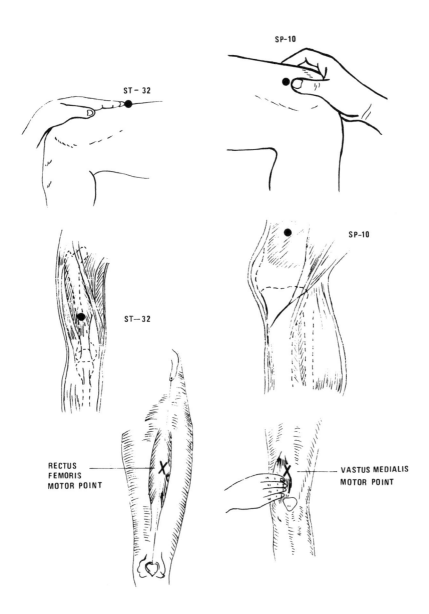

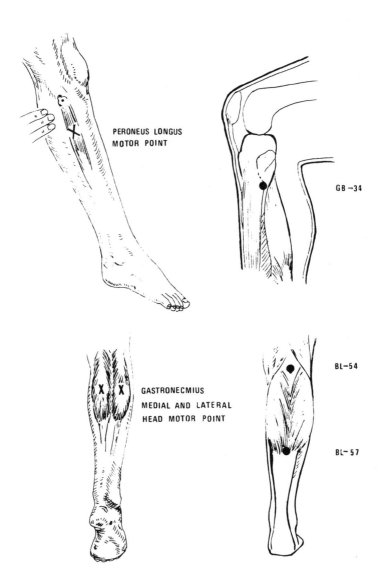

PERONEUS LONGUS
MOTOR POINT

GB -34

GASTRONECMIUS
MEDIAL AND LATERAL
HEAD MOTOR POINT

BL-54

BL-57

T

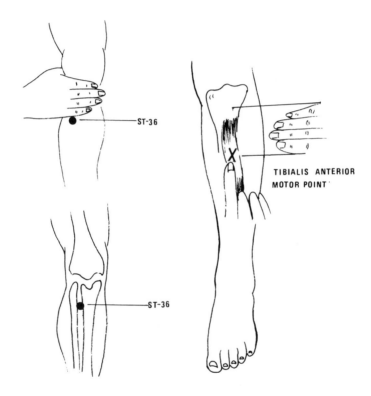

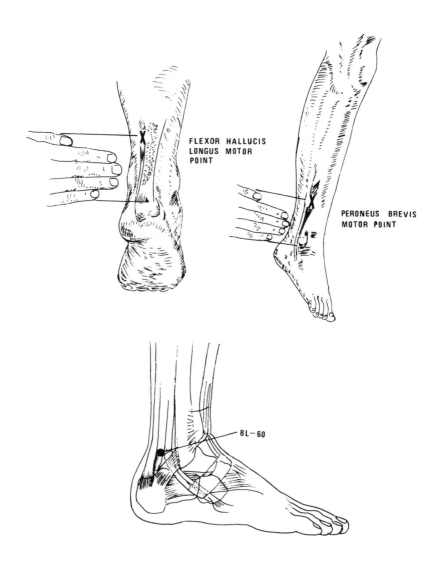

FLEXOR HALLUCIS
LONGUS MOTOR
POINT

PERONEUS BREVIS
MOTOR POINT

BL-60

V

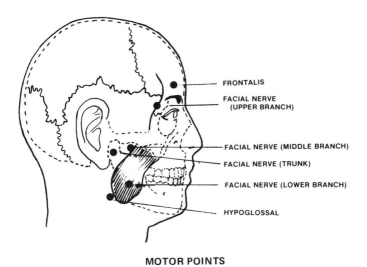

MOTOR POINTS

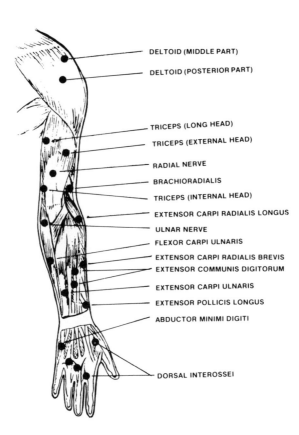

DELTOID (MIDDLE PART)

DELTOID (POSTERIOR PART)

TRICEPS (LONG HEAD)

TRICEPS (EXTERNAL HEAD)

RADIAL NERVE

BRACHIORADIALIS

TRICEPS (INTERNAL HEAD)

EXTENSOR CARPI RADIALIS LONGUS

ULNAR NERVE

FLEXOR CARPI ULNARIS

EXTENSOR CARPI RADIALIS BREVIS

EXTENSOR COMMUNIS DIGITORUM

EXTENSOR CARPI ULNARIS

EXTENSOR POLLICIS LONGUS

ABDUCTOR MINIMI DIGITI

DORSAL INTEROSSEI

MOTOR POINTS

X

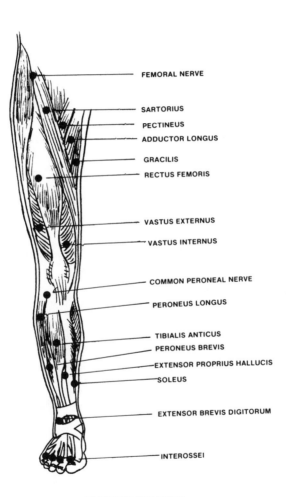

FEMORAL NERVE

SARTORIUS

PECTINEUS

ADDUCTOR LONGUS

GRACILIS

RECTUS FEMORIS

VASTUS EXTERNUS

VASTUS INTERNUS

COMMON PERONEAL NERVE

PERONEUS LONGUS

TIBIALIS ANTICUS

PERONEUS BREVIS

EXTENSOR PROPRIUS HALLUCIS

SOLEUS

EXTENSOR BREVIS DIGITORUM

INTEROSSEI

MOTOR POINTS

Y

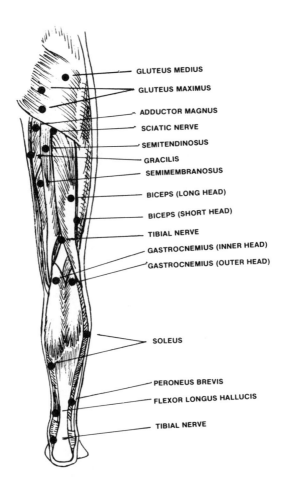

MOTOR POINTS

Z

INDEX

153